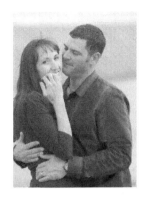 To our family, friends and disease survivors counting every breath with us, we will love you forever.

Jack & Dani

"The Snarky Sarkie & His Sassy Spouse"

We are very excited and honored to announce that after more than 4 years of advocating for total wellness and Sarcoidosis awareness through our radio shows, articles, etc. we now speak at conferences about alternative options outside the prescription! It's time for a paradigm shift and we look forward to what the future holds.

We ARE here for you and will respond to emails. You are not alone in this battle. We look forward to meeting you on our Google hangout events and any time you are crossing through Oregon...let us know.

Cover Photo by Nicole Slater www.indiephotostories.com

Table Of Contents:

Introduction: 3

1: Holistic Health Against All Odds 7

2: Sarcoid...WHAT? The Curve Ball In Our Fairy Tale Life...15

3: Losing Ground – A World Of Uncertainty 20

4: Sarcoidosis Sabbitical - A Fresh Start........................... 30

5: I Tried Everything...Well, Almost Everything! 50

6: The Missing Link Permission to Think Outside the Prescription 58

7: Oxidative Stress, Sarcoidosis, ILDs and 60+ Diseases.... 72

8: We Are What We Absorb So What Should We Eat?..... 91

9:   Anything But Conventional! 124

10: Mind Over Matter Outwitting Sarcoidosis *written by Jack Walker*.. 142

11: Hindsight's Always 20/20!.. 153

12: Resources, Recipes and Links 161

References: 178

Introduction:

Hi! My name is Dani Walker and I am the sassy spouse of Jack Walker, a Sarcoidosis survivor whom I commonly refer to as MY Snarky Sarkie. ☺ Disease is tough but if you've ever been on corticosteroids you know what the "snarky" is all about! This book is a manifestation of the last 9 years of our lives. It all started when Jack was diagnosed with Sarcoidosis – an inflammatory autoimmune related disease[0] in 2004.

According to pubmed.gov Sarcoidosis is a systemic granulomatous disorder of indeterminate origin, manifested by the presence of noncaseating granulomas of virtually any organ system. In layman's terms: There is no known cause or cure for Sarcoidosis; an inflammatory disease which causes granulous tumors to form in any organ system of the body. No cause…no cure…sounds like #@$@! You fill in the #@$@.

We invite you to take a sabbatical before we spur you take action. After all, you must have the "know how" or knowledge before you can implement the plan, right?! It's time for you to relax, put your feet up, rest your bones and recuperate that tired, aching body. As all this information makes your head spin, it still does mine and I've researched, re-read and revised it for over four years now, allow your body to sink into that comfy recliner and rest! Many people with inflammatory/autoimmune disease have benefited greatly by implementing this information and now you can too. I congratulate you and want to thank you for taking your health into your own hands; it's about time!

So, you may be wondering how the heck did we get here? It's a really long story...so let's just start with the day I first heard the word Sarcoidosis. I, Dani, the sassy spouse, will never forget the day that marked a painfully slow erosion of our fairy tale life! It was August 2004, and I immediately blurted out, "Is that worse than Lymphoma?" I never knew such a disease existed and a wave of panic swept over me as I realized we had no idea what we were in for. This book is our saga of overcoming this seemingly incurable disease and a plethora of information on natural options not yet offered by conventional medicine, so you can make a more informed decision for your own health. Never lose hope!

Before we get into our winding path to wellness I want to let you in on a little secret...that "path to wellness" it's complicated! Oh, and another secret...neither of us have any letters behind our names; psychologically unemployable and stubborn as hell...YES, medical professionals...NO. When one person gets sick the entire family feels it...even if they do not talk about it so we are simply real people talking about the good, bad and ugly of dis-ease and the world of options for healing that you may not know exist. We sure didn't!

To my knowledge, Jack and I are the first and only to write about Sarcoidosis from the "Sarkie" and the spouse perspective. As crazy as this sounds, Sarcoidosis has completely transformed our lives for the better but the battle, oh the battle, still rages on. Every day 1,000's of people needlessly suffer from 100's of different disorders.

No matter what disease may be ailing you our goal is to bring a smile and a little laughter (laughter is great medicine) as well as share EVERYTHING we have learned over the last nine years in hopes that your path to healing is much quicker, less confusing, frustrating, expensive, overwhelming and much more HOPEFUL. No two people have lived the same life so the fine print here is: with whatever you choose to implement, results may vary...obviously.

Nine years of information is a lot to take in overnight so please digest at your own pace and MOST IMPORTANTLY, commit to yourself to take this knowledge and put it into action. Do not get analysis paralysis. One step at a time is exactly how we did it!

In the last 9 years we've given Western medicine a go for 3 years, purchased every book, resource guide, subscribed to forums, joined groups, contacted research foundations, etc. etc. We've read Aden Protocol and even though we never used it, we are very familiar with the Marshall Protocol, but never have we found one source that put the pieces together.

This Book has been inspired by many bouts of insomnia, relentless searching fueled by rage and frustration drizzled with literally thousands of emails demanding we put it all together...together, as the "Snarky Sarkie and his Sassy

Spouse!" So there you have it, it is written and dedicated to you. No matter what dis-ease you have, no matter what path you've traveled or multitude of crazy things you've tried...this one's for you!

Know this – we write to give hope! Hope for healing, guidance and encouragement as you travel your own path through this maze called Sarcoidosis (or any sickness). It is all about supporting you in improving your quality of life against all odds! We hope this education beats medication for you as well! We look forward to sharing new alternatives that come our way so be sure to open all emails from life@educationbeatsmedication.com & please share any info or results with us too! Also, this is very important: When you purchased this book you also gained access to 10 exclusive audio interviews. Simply email us your receipt and we will send you login info to access all the audios, videos and future Education Beats Medication events.

Are you ready? Are you ready for us to take you on an arduous journey that actually leads to somewhere? We may not have ALL the pieces and we have yet to find the gold at the end of the rainbow but my "Snarky Sarkie" has been in remission for over 4 years now using the exact methods we share in this book. Best of all, he's not alone, there are hundreds of survivors out there living quality of life over quantity, trading in symptoms and side effects for energy and lifelong solutions. Some choose to use these methods along with medical treatment and others say Sayonara! It's totally your choice.

Chapter 1:   Holistic Health Against All Odds

In this book, Jack and I share our personal journey as well as a road map to the maze of possibilities NOT yet offered by conventional medicine! You know all those late night "google searches" that lead you...right back where you started. ☺ Yeah, we've been there, over and over again actually but not to waste your time or ours, we've cut out all the dead ends and included 10 of my, Dani's, most popular radio show interviews with wellness experts from around the world, covering controversial and edgy yet extremely effective natural methods for total wellness! Controversial and edgy...wouldn't have it any other way. It's like having 10 total wellness experts in your living room!

In 2010, with sheer determination to find real solutions I started a radio show and interviewed naturopaths, leading specialists in functional, oriental, integrative and holistic medicine, neurological chiropractors and more. If I haven't told you yet, I'm tenacious! As you read you will see where we refer you to specific interviews which expand on the topic discussed so be sure to get every ounce of information you can out of this series by listening to every audio! If for some reason you did not get the audios please email life@educationbeatsmedication.com

FYI: Since Jack and I are writing this book together - all of Jack's writing is in **bold** to make it easier for you to know whose perspective you are getting. ☺

When I first talked to Jack about writing a book he said…"I'll wait to see the movie…" ☺ Thus we are in the recording studio now and plan to release our short film "Against All Odds" this Winter!!! I think the blooper reel will be longer than the movie. ☺

Want to know how Jack became his own guinea pig to find a true path to healing which opened us up to a world of alternatives that Western medicine did not offer, has yet to embrace and often criticizes? Keep reading. In this book we share our holistic approach to natural and alternative options that challenged our thoughts, beliefs and certainly the medical community. They still give no credit to any of this "hocus pocus" for Jack's sudden and miraculous remission. Oh well.

In the last 4 ½ years we have witnessed these natural, non-invasive methods help our son with allergies and me with indigestion, migraines and hernias. They have helped people with diabetes, cancer, psoriasis, chronic fatigue (ME), sciatic, Lyme, menopause, scar tissue, arthritis, Trigeminal neuralgia, Sarcoidosis and more live a better quality of life without side effects.

Whether fueled by determination, desperation or a lot of both; this book is for those who dare to think outside the prescription.   You will learn a lot about natural ways to stop tumor formation, suppress certain protein triggers that cause inflammatory disease, relieve coughing, wheezing, and thick phlegm, regain your energy, release stress, breath freely and take back your health. Everything we share can be used in conjunction to medical treatment but of course you should consult your physician before implementing any of this information.

It is important to note that our bodies are meant to be in a state of health, balance and wellness. The symptoms are simply your body screaming at you that "all is NOT well." There are many pieces of the puzzle to wellness and they must ALL fit before it is complete. We know firsthand how exhausting it can be to put the pieces together, ESPECIALLY when so many are missing! For those of us who have grown up with the Western Medicine philosophy, we have been taught that every piece is separate and does not affect the other; thus we go to a different doctor for every ailment.

Once diagnosed, Jack saw a pulmonologist, ENT and rheumatologist for three years. He went to his medical doctors for routine check-ups every 6-9 months. Every six months his pulmonologist would check his heart to see if the granulomas in his mediastinum had changed and perform a lung function test, etc., send him to the ENT who would check the chain of granulomas under his neck and chin, etc. and send him off to the rheumatologist. I think you get the picture.

We have come to know that we are ONE person, ONE body, ONE mind, ONE spirit, ONE universe...maybe we should think that way. This battle to keep disease at bay has lead us to the Eastern medicine philosophy. For thousands of years Chinese have had a deep understanding and respect for foods, herbs and their ability to support our whole body. The basic idea in Chinese medicine is that no single part of the body can be understood without seeking relation to the whole. Thus, finding the underlying cause rather than treating the symptoms is the purpose and the solution. Makes sense! This is the philosophy of a growing movement called Functional Medicine in our Western world and Jack and I welcome it and cannot wait to introduce you to some amazing Functional medicine doctors, Oriental medicine and holistic medicine therapies that we've found on our relentless search for answers.

Chapter 1 Trivia: Listen to the *Surviving Sarcoidosis* audio with Jack & Dani Walker.

What would it be like to pay a doctor to keep you healthy? I think the powers that be (not the doctors) would do whatever it takes to keep us sick and on medicines. But that is just my opinion. ☺

Did you know that historically a Chinese Medicine doctor was paid a retainer to keep their patients healthy? If a patient became sick, the doctor would not be paid until the patient's health was restored. In a similar vein, a doctor that resorted to surgery was considered an inferior doctor. If he/she did their job correctly and helped their clients stay healthy, there would be no need to perform surgery.

What Is Holistic Healing To Me? After much thought, I want to describe what holistic healing is to me (Dani). First of all, I think everyone has the power to heal without medications if they catch the manifestation in time. Physical illnesses are the symptoms of a greater imbalance that may or may not have a root cause in the physical. Having said that, I do respect pharmaceutical medications and feel they have an important role to play in the healing process for some reasons but we should never depend on them for life.

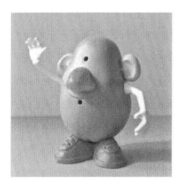 I think it's funny that 'holistic' healing is not spelled whole – but hole – because to me we are "filling" the holes in the whole list! Holistic or "wholistic" healing addresses all parts of the individual, not just the physical aspect of a person where manifested illnesses are most apparent. It does not serve as a band-aid or a one-time fix, but is an ongoing journey of discovery in search of more answers and ultimately living better, being healthier, and striving for wholeness. Our path to holistic health started with a debilitating disease. Some of us have to learn the hard way, I guess. ☺

Because I was so desperate for answers, I did not even realize that I was seeking holistic healing. It became apparent to us that we are all a work in progress when our journey with Jack getting really sick lead our entire family to 'whole healing' – physical healing, mental health and wellness, emotional well-being, and spiritual beliefs and values, where overall wellness AND wholeness became the goal.

My hunger was insatiable; the more I learned the more I questioned and the more willpower I had to make positive, healthy adjustments in my life. Taking this holistic approach involved relentless seeking of tools that would help us attract our desires to live healthy and caused us to take personal responsibility for our own lives, health and lack thereof.

We were initially looking for anything that might help Jack gain some energy and relieve aches and pains but after starting down the path of holistic healing the importance of positive thoughts, tending to relationships, caring for the planet and our environments, having compassion for humankind in general and accepting and tolerating differences among a diverse population of people, became more and more valued in our lives. Disease itself fueled much of this awakening. As Jack got worse, all that was so important, you know, loading the dishwasher right, keeping the car spotless, mowing the lawn in grid fashion so it rivaled the best golf course...all that "important" stuff started to change. Sometimes, in the worst of situations come the best blessings.

The Need for Holistic Healing In Every Life

Discomforts or pains are merely symptoms of an imbalance. The imbalance could be a physical issue, the result of abusing the physical body through an unhealthy diet, lack of exercise, dehydration or too little sleep, years of hard physical labor etc., etc. Or, the imbalance may be the result of mental, emotional, or spiritual needs not being met. No aspect (mind, body, spirit, or emotions) should ever be overlooked in *holistic healing*. After all, we are emotional and electrical beings.

When Jack first started having symptoms of Sarcoidosis (even though we had no idea what it was), my son Trent was also having nasty symptoms that mimicked appendicitis. We were going from one doctor visit for Jack to another for Trent, frantically trying to figure out what WAS wrong with both of them. This continued for almost a year and the final straw for me as a mother was taking Trent to the emergency room (ER) at midnight afraid his appendix was going to burst. After three hours in the ER we left, still with no answer to his stomach aches, swollen lymph nodes, leg cramps, congested cough, headaches, high white blood cell count, etc., etc.

Out of complete frustration and exhaustion we chose to take him to a naturopath and with a simple food allergy test we found out he was allergic to potatoes! Finally, we had an answer to Trent's symptoms after 10 months of expensive doctor visits, drawing blood and invasive poking and prodding. Yahoooo! To this day he is deathly afraid of needles after going through all that. (Listen to "Toxic Food Syndrome" interview with Immuno Labs founder Jeffrey Zavik on Food Intolerance testing and more.)

Our journey into Jacks' medical mystery is to be continued...but for now I am NOT a certified holistic healer, but I believe the patient (i.e. you) has the answers and we are living proof that we can take this approach to wellness and successfully implement it. If you choose to go to a holistic healer remember that it is no different than choosing a medical doctor. YOU decide. If you do not 'agree' find a new one.

The picture is a good demonstration of how every "part" is completely connected.

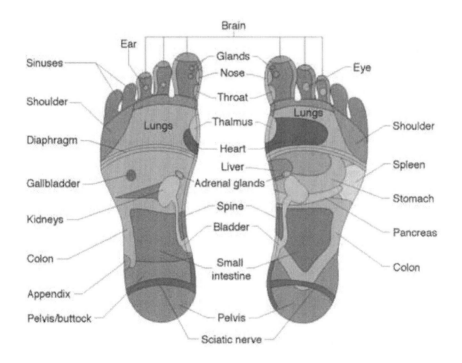

Chapter 2:   Sarcoid...WHAT? The Curve Ball In Our Fairy Tale Life.

Jack and I are risk takers and have always owned our own businesses. By 2003, we had two homes, a successful tree care company, two sons and a "white picket fence." We were living the American Dream and really had created a fairytale life.

Jack was a certified arborist and only 30 years old, in prime physical condition. I cooked everything from scratch, we ate right, exercised, did not smoke, lived in a small town close to family and the world was our oyster! We had just moved into our second home and our tree care business was going better than ever. I worked at UPS 15 hours a week, and got full health benefits for our family at no monthly cost to us. We really felt such blessing on our lives, yet we had no idea how much we took our health for granted. After all, a fairytale is not a fairytale without a lot of struggle, a little drama and some danger. Right?

We discussed Trent's health issues which started around the same time Jacks did. All of Trent's symptoms were completely resolves within a week of cutting potato from his diet! Jack however is another story entirely. During the winter of 2003, at the ripe old age of 31, Jack started showing signs of bronchitis. This was a normal cycle for him so we proceeded with the usual Wellness Formula from the health food store: herbal teas and colloidal silver to try to boost his immune system and fight bronchitis. We used essential oils and even though the bronchitis passed, his lymph nodes under his neck continued to swell; especially the nodes on the right side of his face, under his chin. After a few months of enlarged lymph nodes we started to worry. All I could think was that he may have lymphoma and, if so, we should not waste any more time trying alternatives.

Jack will avoid going to the doctor at all costs, but he finally made an appointment with our primary care physician who ran some blood tests, etc. For the next six plus months he was a medical mystery. His symptoms continued to worsen just as much as my worry! I watched him go from full of energy to no energy at all. He had a raspy cough and complained of aches and pains so intense that his bones hurt. He started working less and less, getting up later and going to bed earlier. Even though he always had a smile on his face, I could tell that whatever "it" was, was taking its toll on us all.

As his lymph nodes continued to grow in size, doctors and specialists ran numerous blood tests, ruling out rare blood diseases, AIDS, etc. They performed a CT-scan, MRI, ultrasounds, upper GI endoscopy, and pulmonary function test. Finally, they thought there may be a possibility that there may be chronic infection in the lymph nodes due to years of having bronchitis, thus, he should have a tonsillectomy in hopes to clear the infection so the lymph could drain. During the procedure in July 2004, a lymph node in his lower neck was removed and a biopsy revealed the final diagnosis...Sarcoidosis.

I am sure you remember the day you were diagnosed as clearly as I do! In our circumstance the very first time we ever heard the word Sarcoidosis was August 14, 2004, the day Jack was diagnosed. All I could think about was "Is that worse than lymphoma?" I am a Mom and worry is second nature. For months I had secretly and mentally prepared myself for "the worst" and in my mind it was lymphoma. Cancer must be the worst...right? I had researched treatment options, alternative therapies etc. and felt like I was prepared for our next step but...Sarcoidosis!?!? A wave of panic washed over me, as I had NO CLUE what we were in for. What is the treatment? What is the disease? What the hell is Sarcoidosis? What do I tell the boys? Will Jack live? Will I be a widow? I am only 29 and we are TOO YOUNG to be dealing with any of this! We should get a second opinion.

I held myself together, but as Sarcoidosis became a part of my reality, all these thoughts and about 10,000 more rushed through my head in a matter of seconds. It was all so surreal. We wanted a diagnosis. We had waited for so long to finally get one and in knowing what he "had" I felt completely lost in an abyss of uncertainty and fear.

Inside I was panicking, rejecting this new information, but I was too afraid to show it. I remember looking at Jack, at his swollen lymph nodes under his neck and wondering, will they ever go away? Will it get worse? Will he ever heal? What the heck is he thinking right now? He eats right, he exercises, he does not smoke, and he is only 31...why is this happening to us? It does not make sense. There has to be a reason…an explanation. I want answers and I want them now! We need a second opinion!

JACK :   I remember clearly. The thought going through my mind was how does one go from healthy and active to having a rare disease with an uncertain outcome? I was at a crossroad: I could either be afraid of dying or really start living.

It was time for me to reprioritize my life, from family, health, diet and where to focus my energy. I shifted my thoughts from spending time building our tree care business to what really mattered: time with family.

Chapter 2 Trivia: Listen to interview *The Epigenetics Of Chronic Illness* with Naturopath Dr. Richard Powell & Neurological Chiropractor Dr Michael Gruttadauria.

Does our environment; where you live, what you eat, breath, drink, do for a living, and expose yourself to, have more to do with your health than your genetics? We say – YES.

- "Aging and disease are 90% environmental and 10% genetic." --Aubrey de Gray, acclaimed Geneticist
- Based on Harvard studies and Genome Mapping, our lifespan potential is 200 years.
- Sarcoidosis knows no cause or cure and has no proof of being hereditary but is most prevalent in Scandanavians and African American women. Why?

- One theory suggests that Sarcoidosis develops when a genetically susceptible person is exposed to specific environmental agents. Although the specific agents are unknown, several organisms, including viruses and bacteria, have been suggested as possible causes. Noninfectious chemicals in the environment, including beryllium, aluminum, and zirconium, can cause lung disease that has features similar to sarcoidosis. [1]

A little medical history on Jack: He had pneumonia as a baby which led to chronic bronchitis every fall which we did our best to treat naturally without antibiotics. Other than this and suffering from heart burn, he was in perfect health...so we thought. He also spent 20+ years of his life in the trees. As a certified arborist he breathed in a lot of fine saw dust while trimming, removing and pruning trees.

We have no proof that either of the above situations played a part in Jack's Sarcoidosis (primarily a lung disease), but we certainly think they are pieces to the puzzle. In addition, my (Dani) four plus years of meeting people with 'Sarc' from around the world and hearing their stories, has led me to completely agree with the above theory. I feel that there are people who are genetically predisposed to Sarcoidosis and due to one or numerous environmental agents, dormant genes are triggered which manifest the dis-ease Sarcoidosis. The challenge is figuring out what these triggers are so you can rid or protect your life from these environmental agents and take back your health.

Chapter 3: Losing Ground In A World Of Uncertainty

"Winning isn't everything, it's the only thing." Vince Lombardi

Okay, so we got the diagnosis out of the way...now what? I wondered if Jack was the only person on the planet with Sarcoidosis and I am sure he thought the same. All the answers to our questions were still a mystery and we were told the best option was drugs...prednisone, to be exact.

After Jack was diagnosed, he started to see three specialists and continued to see his M.D.'s (Medical Doctors). He was initially prescribed a whopping 80mg of prednisone a day, the #1 prescribed medication for inflammatory diseases like Sarcoidosis! After a week he had gained 10+ pounds and was a walking time bomb. He is a pretty high energy guy by nature so prednisone did not help any.

JACK: After gaining that prednisone weight, I started riding my bike to no avail. I went from 220 to 270+ in less than a year. I tried cutting out red meat, alcohol, sugar, etc. but nothing worked. When I asked my Doctor what I could do to lose the weight he responded, "When you are on this drug there is nothing you can do."

I will never forget the day my Mom showed up with a book of information she had printed for us to read and demanded that we go see a specialist in California. I adore her for how much she cares and worries about us all. She had stayed up all night searching for solutions to Sarcoidosis online and was in complete panic because of the information she found. I know she just felt helpless and wanted to do whatever she could but for me it was all too much, too fast.

We had just found out Jack had Sarcoidosis and none of us really even understood what that meant. Within two weeks he was driving two hours away to see three specialists, Mom was handing me a ton of scary information, and I just wanted to go back to bed. Wake me up when the devastation is over!

As the first year of disease progressed the emotional stress took its' toll and Jack and I were not communicating this to each other. The slow erosion of our lives had begun. What medications and check-ups were not taking, frustration and aggravation would. I was going through my day with a smile and acting as though all was well, even though uncertainty had overtaken my every thought. I was ruled by unanswered "What ifs".

Jack was edgy, in tons of pain and always tired, thus the nickname "Snarky Sarkie".   You never really knew how he was going to respond to anything. Within six months he went from working 50-60 hour weeks climbing trees every day, to barely being able to climb 3-4 hours once or twice a week. He had gained almost 60 pounds, and he was feeling the financial burden and emotional pressure of not being able to provide for us.

As a wife, I did not want to complain to him because he was the one with Sarcoidosis. Who am I to whine and cry when he was the one who was actually sick? As a mom there was no way in hell I was going to show even a crack of concern for the future. The boys were only 4 and 8 and I had to hold it together, taking on a "No big deal" attitude, I let them know that Dad was going to be okay. We would all get through this.

Not to bother Dad, the boys were relying more and more on me for everything. Every time I turned around they were asking this and that and needing me for something. I recall daily when they both be at me with "Mom, can you help me? Mom, how do you do this? Mom, come here. Moooooommmmm." I did the best I could, but out of complete exhaustion I yelled, "You have a Dad that can help you, too!" The shower and car were my safe havens. "I'm going for a drive" or "I'm taking a shower" were codes for "I am about to lose it!"

Often times I was cold and insensitive towards Jack. He would wake up in the morning and say something like, "I haven't even gotten up yet and I feel like I have been hit by a Mack truck." Without understanding or empathy for what he was going through I would hold in my anger and frustration and then respond with, "Well aren't you going to work today?" Watching our business and main source of income slowly dissolve right along with Jack's health was unbearable. I rarely thought about what it would be like to have a growth on my face. How I would act if I was exhausted and in pain all the time or if I had gained 60 pounds in a year! I had not thought about how this

emotionally affected Jack. Yet, when I have one small zit on my chin I freak out and do everything I can to hide it!
It was not until he actually started to heal that I met other people with Sarcoidosis who were on 13+ medications and disability, needed lung transplants, etc., etc., that I finally started to grasp the severity of what he had been going through.

I share all this with you in hopes that it brings more understanding and compassion between couples who are dealing with a spouse who is battling disease. I may not be the only one who has a strange way of dealing with a sick spouse. It was not because I did not care, but more because I was scared to death and just did not want to tell him. I often forgot Sarcoid was the enemy, not him.

Every night I went to bed thinking about Sarcoidosis and asking God to heal Jack. Every morning I woke up thankful that he was still with us and wondering how we were going to physically, financially, emotionally and spiritually get through it. A "miraculous remission" did not seem to be in the cards.

Because I worked at UPS, we had full health benefits that paid 80% of everything, thank goodness. After three years and $100,000+ of testing and treatment costs, we still had more than $8,000 in medical debt left to pay off after years of monthly payments. Even though the bucket truck and all the equipment sat in the field, our business was all but done. Jack was on six different medications for everything from GERD to Sarcoidosis and he was sick and tired of feeling like he knew more about this disease than his doctors.

JACK: At this point I started losing hope. I was depressed about having this mystery disease. As far as I knew, there was no getting off of prednisone and no way to combat the side effects; as well as the fact that it was not doing anything to help my Sarcoidosis.

For more than 2 1/2 years I had been taking 40+ mg a day and it did not shrink the granulomas on my face, around my heart or in my lungs. I am so high energy that prednisone actually had a reverse affect and caused depression.

A few of the many visits to my assortment of doctors really stand out to me:

At one appointment my MD told me that the tumors under my chin were fibrocystic and would most likely never go away. On another visit, after cycling for three years, I was told that due to the prolonged prednisone use my thyroid was damaged and I would never lose the weight. (I refuse to give up and to this day I've only got 15 more pounds to go!)

Since I was told the fibrocystic tumors in my lymph nodes would never go away, I was adamant with my ENT/plastic surgeon that he remove the granulous lymph nodes under the right side of my chin because I felt that it was hideous and so many people did a double take in passing. They looked at me like it was a little alien head poking out.☹ The ENT informed me that there is a facial nerve, which if cut, would cause permanent facial paralysis and it was one of the most risky surgeries, thus he refused to perform it.

On yet another visit to my MD, I was told that I needed to take Lipitor because my cholesterol was border line high due to long term prednisone use. At this time I was only 34 and could foresee that this was going to be the 'prescription gauntlet' that I was no longer willing to run. I was done with the direction of Westernized medicine. I refused Lipitor and started to wean myself off prednisone. Doctors warned that this could be dangerous after prolonged use but I was at the end of my proverbial rope. I was just DONE. Always consult your physician before making any changes with your medications. I say this because I don't want to lead you astray or get sued by the FDA.

I saw my pulmonologist one last time and straight up asked him, "What's the difference between the lymph nodes and scar tissue in my lungs and the lymph nodes in Bernie Mac or Reggie White's lungs? Will it kill me, like it killed them?" He responded with, "We hope it burns out."

I knew all my doctors and specialists had my best interest at heart but this was a turning point for me that made me take my life into my own hands and open my mind to alternative options. I had to do some serious soul searching. I went from being fit, athletic and strong with no physical limitations, to being physically incapacitated

and on a drug that was possibly worse for me than the disease. I could either fight or give up and become the disease or overcome the disease. Winning was the only option.

When Jack told me that he was not going back to the specialists and was going to wean himself off prednisone, I was worried but understood. Our bodies are biochemically very, different and what works for one may not work for another. The prednisone did not take away any inflammation. He had been on it for almost three years and was at the point where he could no longer tell the difference between the symptoms of Sarcoidosis and the side effects of the medications. His lymph nodes never shrunk at all and all his specialists could say was, "We hope it burns out." Then they informed him that the swollen lymph nodes had become fibrocystic and even if the Sarc did burn out, they would NEVER go back to their normal size. Oh Boy, did we prove that theory wrong!

Jack was done following a path that led to more medications, more side effects and less quality of life. I could not blame him. Our own journey to finding lasting help without side effects had begun and regardless of the results, we were more than ready.

Even though we did not know where to start, 18 months later, all of Jack's lymph nodes were back to their normal size. He had no signs or symptoms of Sarcoidosis, was completely off all medicines and in his own words he felt like he was 19 again! That is even better than before Sarcoid. ☺

Chapter 3 Trivia: Do not forget to believe and breathe!

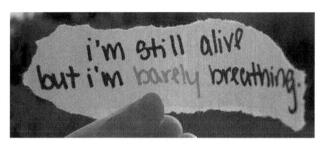

How important is oxygen? Silly question but one most of us don't even consider until we are short of breath.

The average American has 21,600 breaths every 24 hours (15 breaths per min X 60 min X 24 hours). The breathing process is the foundation of all brain function and 12 energy systems of the body. The respiratory system feeds our cardiovascular system and supports our digestive and lymphatic systems: two systems paramount to processing food and the removal of toxins and imbalances from the body. Breathing is also the only physiological function that can be controlled.[2]

1. **70% of waste is eliminated through your lungs:** *The Tao of Breathing* by Dennis Lewis, states that "70% of our body's waste products are eliminated via our lungs and the rest through the urine, skin and feces." When the efficiency of our lungs is reduced due to poor breathing, less oxygen is available to our cells. It slows down the flow of blood which carries wastes from the kidneys and lungs. Our lymphatic

system which fights off viral and bacterial invaders is weakened, along with causing a slower digestive process.

2. **Your breath is the first thing to respond in your body:** Your breath will respond and adjust according to what you are thinking, feeling, observing, hearing, tasting, touching, sensing or experiencing at the time. It is intimately connected to your physical, emotional and spiritual state.

3. **Check the depth of your inhale:** This is a great place to start developing a greater understanding of your breath by focusing on the depth of your inhale. A full inhale should fill your lungs and expand your abdomen. Place your hands onto either side of your lower ribs. Feel them expand with each inhale. Then place your hands onto your belly and feel it rise and fall with each breath.

4. **Breathing Technique:** Place the tongue on the roof of the mouth; this accesses the right side of the brain, the intuition, and the feeling part of the brain. Inhale with the tongue on the roof of the mouth. Picture white light coming up both meridians, meeting on the roof of the mouth. Now visualize the breath traveling down the whole GI tract with the exhale out the tailbone. Begin again, inhale white light for 7 counts, hold for 4 counts, and exhale for 8 counts.

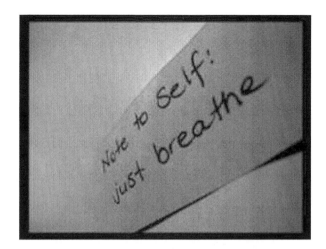

5. **Breath In, Breath Out:** The neck is the Emotional Bridge between the brain and the heart! If you always have neck pain or tight shoulders, implement this breathing technique a couple of times a day, 3-5 breaths at a time and witness the result. Putting this into practice can lower stress, increase energy and strengthen your immune system!

Chapter 4: Sarcoidosis Sabbitical - A Fresh Start

"A new scientific truth is not usually presented in a way to convince its opponents. Rather, they die off, and a rising generation is familiarized with the truth from the start." — Max Planck

So how did Jack do it? That is what you really want to know, and we are so excited to share. But first, I have to tell you a story about what I like to call our "Sarcoidosis Sabbatical." To help us get into the right mindset to embark on our new journey, we needed a break from Sarcoidosis first.

Jack was on 40mg a day of prednisone when he started weaning down. We were on year four of surviving Sarcoidosis and both of us were feeling lost and exhausted. He had come to a crossroad and decided to take the path less traveled but we needed some rest before maneuvering uncharted territory. Summer was coming, the boys would be out of school and at the time, I was working three hours a day at UPS. We were in a space of life where all the "logical and responsible" decisions we had ever made seemed meaningless.

Every day was a blessing and we wanted to make the best of each one, so I did what any sane person would do. I quit my job! Health insurance, or sickness insurance, as I like to call it, was not going to pay for any of the alternatives Jack would try, so why stay and lose precious time with my husband? The future was uncertain and time together was all we were living for.

I remember how many people could not believe that I would quit such a great job. I, too, was having a difficult time believing it. After all, jobs are hard to come by in such a small town. Many people disagreed with Jack's choice to stop treatment, yet with all the uncertainties of what our future held, we embarked on this journey together. I know now that it was divine guidance that led us to make such seemingly irresponsible decisions.☺

We wanted to spend time doing fun things as a family, so Jack sold his motorcycle and we bought a PURPLE (color for Sarcoidosis) raft! We sold one of our homes and we were off…for the summer, that is! No 'Sarcoidosis speak.' We just pretended like Sarc was no more and spent the summer rafting, camping and chilling with the boys. This was 'healing balm for our sore spirits' and marked the beginning of the end of erosion; a time for rebuilding what was lost. Yes, Jack was still tired, aching and struggling with Sarcoidosis but it was a marvelous summer, a much needed reprieve and memories we continue to think of daily.

As summer quickly came to an end Jack and I started talking about what to do, where to start and how. We knew we were going to take a turn down 'alternative lane' but there were so many options. Where should we start? We decided to simply take a step! With a pinch of blind faith, a dash of hope and several books like *Eat Right for Your Blood Type* and *The Acid Alkaline Diet,* we took off down the trail.

We had lots of input from friends and family. Everyone had an idea of what Jack should try, take, do, etc., and he was open to most of it.

Here is the list of the many different holistic healing options Jack used over the next 18-month period:

Ayurveda medicine	natural diet
herbal remedies	homeopathy
acupuncture	naturopathic medicine
bodywork	energy-based therapies
prayerful intention	Chinese medicine
exercise	nutritional supplements

Remember, we are not Sarcoidosis experts, doctors, or nutritionists, so our path was not a clean, well thought out, step-by-step process. It was more a 'throw everything that comes our way at Sarcoidosis' and see what works. Wait a minute! That is not much different than Western medicine.☺

It was a complete experiment of stubborn proportions and Jack was a very committed guinea pig. He always used to say, "I would rather be my own guinea pig than someone else's." Of course, we had no idea that this crazy, windy path would lead to remission and a life of helping people overcome disease and the debt caused by it, but amazing things happen for those who do not lose hope!

For months after he refused further medical treatment, he was trying diets, supplements, cleanses, etc., and feeling no improvement, but he did not give up...he stayed the course one step at a time and you must do the same. It takes your body years to manifest dis-ease and it will take time to repair it. We really feel that it is important for us to share Jack's path as precisely as possible so you can see that his recovery was not overnight (around 18 months), nor effortless, but took great commitment and opened us up to a world of amazing people, products, support and guidance.

Jack: I knew I could not keep doing what I was doing and expect a different result. It took several months to safely wean myself off 40mg of prednisone a day, but by August 2007, I had finally done it. Almost three years to the date of my diagnosis.

Even though we all have Sarcoidosis, our lives and circumstances are very individual so I want to paint a picture of my daily environment before and during allopathic (Western medicine) treatment.

Our Family's Daily lifestyle: Our normal eating habits have always been rather good. We do not drink sodas. We grow food in our family garden, buy farm fresh eggs from a friend and grass-fed, organic beef from another friend. We eat meat as a side dish rather than the main dish. We have never been much for dairy and drink coconut or almond milk. I won't even get into what is in the dairy products you find in grocery stores right now but I will say the dairy causes mass inflammation within the body and I once read a study that said 70% of Americans are lactose intolerant and don't even know it. We do not do soy

either. Soy and corn are the two most genetically modified crops and soy is an estrogen mimic which has been linked to causing boys to become more feminine and girls to mature faster and increase the risk of certain cancers. Most of the time, Dani cooks from scratch and one of the great things about living in a small rural area is that there are no fast food restaurants! Thank goodness because we do not need the temptation. ☺

I count my blessings that my Sarcoidosis has not been completely debilitating and I could always ride my bike for mental escape and some exercise. I did go through months of great pain that prevented me from exercising, but most of the time I was able to at least get out a couple times a week.

The air is clean and life is at a much slower pace here in northeast Oregon. We filter our drinking water. This is VERY important. I am a HUGE water snob and will not even drink *any* water that is not filtered. I'm known for saying "You can either buy a filter or be a filter, period!" So please, please, please buy a filter. Yes, I'm begging, Dani would call it demanding, however you want to look at it, your cells will thank me.

Dani has always been conscious of the fact that whatever we put on our skin ends up going down the drain, into our waterways, and possibly polluting the Earth. She has done her best to buy bisphenol-free (BPA) containers, glass jars, etc., and 100% toxin-free toothpaste, shampoo, lotions, detergents and cosmetics.

We do miss a few wonderful conveniences by living so remotely: We only have one main grocery store so "What you see is what you get" has something to be desired. Fresh, organic produce is VERY seasonal and expensive, but we manage by canning and freezing as much as we can. You may have many great options where you live but we are two hours from Costco and five hours from a Whole Foods or Trader Joe's. As much as we love to support local business, some things you just can't find here. Thus online ordering has really supported our lifestyle change. Many places offer discounts and free shipping. We order several things like flax seed, hemp powder, coconut flour, etc., from Amazon and we absolutely recommend Azure Standard, a family owned business, where we have found the best prices for organic bulk foods, toxin-free personal care, etc. (See Chapter 12 for these resources and more)

Please keep in mind that this was already our daily lifestyle, so Jack only had to make minor changes to his diet, hydration, exercise, etc. If you are reading and feeling overwhelmed, please know that you can start with one thing. What can you do today to start on the path to health? Look at it like this: add one good thing for a multitude of great benefits. Commit to continue on this path for at least 90 days. If all you can do right now is commit to taking one step every 90 days, then do it. Exchange soda for water and choose one more thing to change after that. It may not sound like a lot but if you do this, you will be amazed at how much better you feel and how much more willing you are to make more life adjustments. It's pretty cool to see how addicting it is to live a limitless life! Especially for those of us who've been confined by dis-ease.

I feel that what holds us back from really taking charge of our health is that we "think" we have to go raw, vegan, exercise three hours a day, drink 15 gallons of water every day (exaggeration), cut out all the chocolate, chips, pop, alcohol, candy, coffee, etc., and never indulge again. This is not the case, not our case anyway. We do our best to find healthy alternatives to all of these things, but of course, every now and then, we indulge. I cannot stress enough that we are real people. We eat a pizza once in a while. Should we? No, but we still do. We stop at In and Out when we are traveling. It is Jack's favorite burger place! ☺ Sometimes we pay for it by feeling yucky after but it's a great reminder of just how sensitive our bodies are and how good it feels to feel good.

The entire reason we have traveled this path is so we can LIVE life and enjoy it so please know that you can, too. Yes, you may have to pass up that Coke or Trix for breakfast every morning, but that does not mean you can never have them again. Everything in moderation, quality of life is what we are after and it is going to take some effort!

Ok, back to the story...It was our summer sabbatical and we took full advantage of it but three months goes by fast and reality hit home quickly. We made the difficult decision to sell all our tree care equipment and really succumb to the fact that Jack's arborist career was over (or so we thought).

We needed an income so I did what I said I would never do and started managing our family's restaurant. Bye bye life, hello paycheck. Do not get me wrong, I am forever grateful to have had that option but it was 24/7.

Now it was time to deal with Sarcoidosis! Jack was finally weaned off prednisone so we thought that cleansing his body would help get rid of any lingering prednisone and give him a fresh start. Our first stop was the local health food store to find some cleansing options.

We chose Renew Life CleanseSMART for two simple reasons. First, the owner highly recommended it. Second, Jack really wanted a slow, safe cleanse in hopes of ridding his body of any lasting prednisone and creating a more alkaline environment for long-term health. CleanseSMART seemed to be the best option available. It is a two-part, 30 day, advanced herbal cleansing program. It is formulated to stimulate the detoxification process of the body's seven channels of elimination: the liver, lungs, colon, kidneys, blood, skin, and lymphatic system.

Since cleansing is almost a lost art in America we really knew little about it other than it made sense and seemed like a good idea. We've since learned a lot and incorporate cleansing into our life every 6-12 months. If you are considering a cleanse please listen to the audio "How To Cleanse Safely" with Dani & Dr. Richard Powell first. This audio is a wealth of information on how to have a successful cleanse without nasty side effects. When cleansing toxins are flushed into your bloodstream within

48 hours after starting a cleanse. Ridding your body of stored toxins too quickly can be very dangerous, especially if you are on multiple medications. There are many different options for cleansing. A good 5-7 day juice cleanse can be extremely effective but you should have a professional advising you.

During Jack's cleanse, as toxins were pulled from his cells and flushed into his blood stream to be excreted, during the second week he did experience some headaches, nausea and fatigue. Hydration is key to cleansing. Keeping properly hydrated can relieve these symptoms and increase the cleansing effect. By the end of the 30-day cleanse, he had lost a few pounds of the prednisone weight and he has remained completely regular ever since. This may be TMI (too much information) but we should all be using the bathroom 2-3 times a day, within 30-45 minutes after each meal.

Again, for those of you who are on many medications, please consult your physician before considering a cleanse/detox and work with a professional during your cleanse. When we were searching for cleansing options the 'Hope To Heal' home cleanse was not yet available but this is the cleanse we now do. You will find a link to the *Hope To Heal* book, a step-by-step home cleanse with DVD for easy and complete instruction, in the resource section of chapter 12.

The Concept Of Cleansing: Listen to "The Lost Art Of Cleansing" with Dr. Laurel Sander

Think of your blood as the streams of your body carrying nutrients to every cell, organ, and tissue, then taking toxins and by-products to the excretory organs. The 22 feet from the mouth opening to the seven sphincters muscles of the rectum is the main river of the human body. This is an excretory organ that descends and excretes the toxins and byproducts.

The human body is a filtration system. Every molecule of nutritious food, water and unidentified food products that are ingested must be absorbed through the mucous membrane of the intestines which then travel directly to the liver, the filter for the blood. The clean blood with essential nutrients nourishes and regenerates all organs and tissues. The liver dumps the dirty, leftover byproducts into the gall bladder. Then the gall bladder dumps its byproducts into the top of the small intestine. This completes a full circle: intestines, liver, gall bladder, and back to the intestines.

The top of the small intestine is called the solar plexus. It is the second largest nerve plexus in the body. The spleen, stomach and pancreas all start the digestion process and deliver the "food chime" to the small intestine where it will be absorbed into the body.

The lymphatic system has little pumps all over the body. They pump one direction -- up. The lymph system cleans out the soft tissues, the muscles, tendons and ligaments. In order for the lymphatic pumps to pump debris up, you must move! The lymph will not work if you are stagnant. The most effective movement to get your lymph to pump is cross crawl movement like walking or bouncing on a rebounder (a small indoor trampoline). So the lymph system is busy cleaning out the byproducts of the muscular function and injuries like lactic acid, uric acid, prussic and oxalic acid, enema fluid and dead red-blood cells. Yuck! Then the lymph system pumps and cleanses out the muscles and dumps these byproducts into the venous system (veins) and then loops back into the intestines and pushes the waste out...eventually.

The appendix is a finger-shaped filter that is located below the ileocecal valve between the small and large intestine. Its function is to gather heavy debris and toxins, like an oil filter. It used to be that each spring when people naturally cleansed, the appendix was able to dump the accumulation acquired over the course of a year.

Cleansing and detoxification are almost a lost knowledge in the land of abundance and convenience but the fact is....

Your body wants to cleanse itself.

In fact, it is working around the clock to clear toxins it is exposed to every day. Your body was made to work perfectly on natural foods and in a natural lifestyle. As we talked about earlier in the chapter, we are simply not equipped to process the huge volume of toxic chemicals we are currently exposed to every day in our air, water, personal care and food supply. Thus, cleansing is where Jack started. He wanted a "fresh start" to build a good foundation for healing and recovery.

As you read the rest of this book it chronicles our story and study of alternative options for true healing. Be sure to refer to Chapter 12 and the audio interviews for more information on alternative options for helping your body heal seemingly incurable diseases.

We've covered cleansing in detail but I think two of the most important things you can do for the immediate health of you and your families is rid your bathroom of toxic products and buy a water filter! We are one of the first generations to be raised and live in such massive pollution. There are more than 100,000 toxic chemicals in our environment today, that did not even exist 50 years ago.[3] We drink plastic molecules, use toxic chemicals on our skin found in lotions and potions, inhale and ingest particles from fertilizers and pesticides and eat microwaved foods. Throw in petroleum products, hydrogenated fats, lots of synthetic hormones and synthetic prescription medications and you have a chemical stew that has been "nourishing" our body for years! This is the environment we may live in but we can and must do something about it if we really want to be healthy and heal. Our environment is within our power to control, or more accurately, our willpower to control. You already buy toothpaste, shampoo, deodorant, cosmetics, shave gel, lotion, etc. as the bottles empty, replace them with toxin-free products. You already drink water, now drink pure water that your body can assimilate!

So why is it so important to go toxin free?

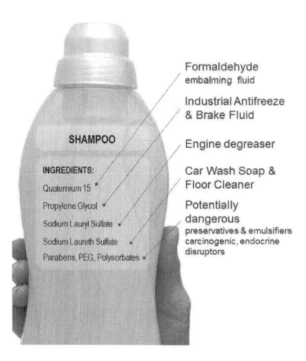

Formaldehyde embalming fluid

Industrial Antifreeze & Brake Fluid

Engine degreaser

Car Wash Soap & Floor Cleaner

Potentially dangerous preservatives & emulsifiers carcinogenic, endocrine disruptors

SHAMPOO

INGREDIENTS:
Quaternium 15
Propylene Glycol
Sodium Lauryl Sulfate
Sodium Laureth Sulfate
Parabens, PEG, Polysorbates

"We look good, we smell good, and we have just exposed ourselves to 200 different chemicals a day through cosmetics."...U.S. News and World Report

"No law requires manufacturers to list the exact ingredients on the package label." Debra Lynn Dadd, Home Safe Home (Tarcher-Putnam, 1997).

"The EU Cosmetics Directive (76/768/EEC) was revised in January 2003 to ban 1,328 chemicals from cosmetics; the U.S. FDA has banned or restricted only 11." The Campaign for Safe Cosmetics

Check out all your shampoos, conditioners, lotions, hair dyes, fingernail polish, polish remover, cosmetics, sun screens, toothpaste, mouth washes, etc., for toxins and chemicals that are being absorbed through your skin and hair follicles. Your skin and hair are a direct source into your blood supply. Try rubbing a piece of garlic on the bottom of your foot, how long does it take to taste it? Look for any numbers like red dye #6. Also, be aware of isopropyl alcohol, parabens, sodium laurel sulfate, Dioxin, EDTA, PEG, phthalates, and triclosan, just to name a few.

When different ingredients are combined, they have the ability to create new (undisclosed) ingredients like dioxin, commonly found in beef, fish, shampoos and skin creams. In addition to cancer, exposure to dioxin can also cause severe reproductive and developmental problems (at levels 100 times LOWER than those associated with its cancer causing effects). **Dioxin is well-known for its ability to damage the immune system** and interfere with hormonal systems. Many studies link this chemical to the reason for low progesterone levels in women. Be sure to listen to the "Toxic Times How It's Made" audio to learn more about what these chemicals are and how they affect our health as well as our environment.

One of the main reasons women are more toxic than men is because we actually take care of ourselves. We think all these chemical ridden products will stop wrinkles, soften skin, make our hair shinier, when in reality they cause us to age more quickly because of the numerous and dangerous chemicals. I ask you to do me one favor and go to www.skindeep.com and enter the name of some of your favorite gels, lotions, shave gels, makeup, and shampoos to see just how toxic they really are. You will be as shocked as I was!

As we all know, skin is the largest organ on our body! Everything we put on our skin soaks into other organs and tissues. In my opinion the toxins found in household cleaners and personal care products are the #1 reason for chronic autoimmune diseases. Think about how many times you have used lotion in your life? How many times you have brushed your teeth, washed your body, etc. Every time we do these routine things we are exposing our brain, liver, lungs, heart, and blood to hundreds of toxic chemicals that cause everything from respiratory problems to seizures!

Becoming aware of this, for the health of my family, I was compelled to stop supporting the companies that make these toxic products and go toxin-free. Jack and I encourage you to do the same. It is sad but true that our real power to make positive change is in our wallet! We each work our butts off to make ends meet and then we go give that hard earned money to large corporations who do not care about our health and obviously the FDA is not going to step in as the European Union (EU) has. Instead, we must be aware and start putting our money into our own health and the health of future generations. If you are going to buy personal care and cleaning products, buy them from companies that make toxin-free products. If you want to make your own, know that the ingredients are inexpensive, effective and safe and the recipes are simple.

Lemon is an excellent disinfectant. Vinegar cleans better than most chemical astringents. Baking soda can be used to clean, scrub, deodorize and more! We use Dr. Bronners and buy it by the gallon from Azure Standard. It is toxin-free and can be used for everything from washing cars and clothes to hair (Refer to Chapter 12).

We have covered many reasons why it is imperative to go toxin-free, now let us talk about the importance of filtering your water. There are so many pollutants in our drinking water: chlorine, fluoride, lead, arsenic, plastics, etc. Independent studies in such journals as *Reviews of Environmental Contamination and Toxicology*; *Environmental Health Perspectives*; *American Journal of Public Health*; and *Archives of Environmental and Occupational Health*, as well as, reports published by the National Academy of Sciences, suggest that millions of Americans become sick each year from drinking contaminated water, with maladies from upset stomachs to cancer and birth defects.

As Jack said earlier, he is a total water snob and I, Dani, will indeed agree. No matter how thirsty he may be he won't drink the water unless it's filtered! Since the day I met Jack, we've had water filters for our home, our water bottles, camping, you name it. Our last one was a solid carbon block countertop unit that wore out after 13 years of use and after tons of research we chose a Big Berkey filter. It is rated #1 for removing volatiles, fluoride, arsenic, microbes, etc. etc. I was not a fan of it because it sits on the kitchen counter and takes up space but after my first drink, I became a believer. As Jack always says "You can either buy a filter or BE a filter."

How Hydrated Are We?

Hydration is the first key to health and water really is the elixir of life. The earth is 2/3 water, the human body is a replica of the earth, and Humans are 66% or 2/3 water when we are born.

- FACT: Dehydration is the #1 cause of death in our elderly! Our nations' population of 70-80 years old are only 12-17% water when they die – chronic dehydration!

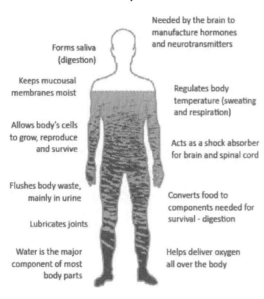

Needed by the brain to manufacture hormones and neurotransmitters

Forms saliva (digestion)

Keeps mucousal membranes moist

Regulates body temperature (sweating and respiration)

Allows body's cells to grow, reproduce and survive

Acts as a shock absorber for brain and spinal cord

Flushes body waste, mainly in urine

Converts food to components needed for survival - digestion

Lubricates joints

Water is the major component of most body parts

Helps deliver oxygen all over the body

- Water molecules must be pure and line up in single file to be absorbed by a cell or a herniated disk.
- Pure water is absorbed 5-7 times faster than polluted water, a process that can take 48 hours.
- It can take two days to filter pure water from a soda. Do not let media fool you...corn syrup cannot replace water!

- Use ice water sparingly. Your stomach must heat all drink and food up to 98.6 degrees before it can start to digest it.
- Drink water between meals and add fresh squeezed lemon to alkalize your body.
- Gradually increase the amount of daily water as the urination increases.
- Add electrolytes - we are made of salt-water not bottled water!
- Take mineral supplements, add sea salt on food, take Epsom salt baths. Soaking for 15 minutes in a hot bath is a great way to re-hydrate.

Every time my boys come to me and say, "I have a headache," my first response is, "Drink some water." Many times we take aspirin when we really should drink water. Our lungs are 83% water and the brain is 80% water. When dehydration occurs, the body goes into a regulatory rationing system; the brain and organs receive the water first, and some cells receive just enough to survive. As these dehydrated cells stick together and thicken, they look like raisins on a blood test.

How much water should you drink every day?

We need a half ounce of water for every pound that we weigh. If you weigh 150 pounds, drink 75 ounces a day or 30 millimeters per kilograms of body weight. For every cup of coffee, alcoholic beverage or soda, add one more cup of water to compensate for their dehydrating effects.

Chapter 4 Trivia: What are your medications depriving you of?

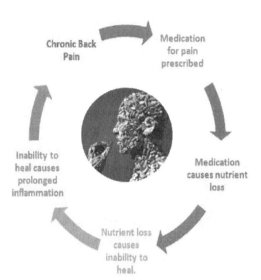

Chronic Back Pain

Medication for pain prescribed

Medication causes nutrient loss

Nutrient loss causes inability to heal.

Inability to heal causes prolonged inflammation

Allopathic (Western Medicine) prescriptions can cause dehydration, as well as, depletion of valuable nutrients our bodies need in order to heal. This only further complicates symptoms and can add to more dis-ease.

Antacids, such as, Pepcid, Tagamet and Zantac, deplete our bodies of vitamins B12, D, Folic Acid, Calcium, Iron and Zinc.

Prevacid and Prilosec depletes our body of vitamin B12.

Antibiotics, such as, general aminoglycosides (gentomycin, neomycin, streptomycin), cephalosporins, penicillins, deplete our bodies of B and K vitamins, and friendly beneficial intenstinal bacteria.

Tetracyclines depletes our bodies of calcium, zinc, magnesium, iron, and vitamin B6.

Anti-diabetics such as Micronase and Tolinase, deplete our bodies of co-enzyme Q10. glucophage, vitamin B12, and folic acid.

Anti-depressants such as: Adapin, Aventyl, Elavil, Tofranil, Pamelor, Sinequan, and
Norpramin, depletes our bodies of vitamin B12 and co-enzyme Q10.

Anti-Inflammatories such as Aspirin and Salicylates, depletes our bodies of vitamin C, folic acid, iron and potassium.

Advil, Aleve, Anaprox, Dolobid, Feldene, Lodine, Motrin, Naprosyn, Orudis, and Relafen, depletes our body of folic acid. Betamethasone, Cortisone, Dexamethasone,

Hydrocortisone, **Methylprednisolone, and Prednisone**, depletes our bodies of vitamin C and D, folic acid, calcium, magnesium, potassium, selenium, and zinc.

Cardiovascular drugs such as Apresoline depletes our bodies of vitamin B6 and co-enzyme Q10. Catapres and Aldomet depletes our bodies of co-enzyme Q10. Corgard, Inderal, Lopressor, Betapace, Tenormin, Sectral and Blocadren depletes our bodies of co-enzyme Q10 and melatonin.

Cholesterol lowering agents (statins), such as: Lescol, Lipitor, Mavacor, Zocor, Pravachol and Crestor depletes our bodies of co-enzyme Q-10. Colestid and Quetran depletes our bodies of vitamins A, B12, D, E, K, beta carotene, folic acid, and iron.

Chapter 5: I Tried Everything…Well, Almost Everything!

"I may have Sarcoidosis but it does NOT have me." Jack Walker

I know that last chapter was an eye opener for many of you but we are only 1/3 of the way through the book so get ready for us to broaden your horizons even more! To recap, after Jack refused any further medical treatment he immediately started to wean himself off of prednisone. This is not a quick, fun or simple process as there can be many negative withdrawals during the tapering process, especially when you taper off to quickly. This is because prednisone is similar to cortisol, a hormone naturally made by your adrenal glands. If you take prednisone for more than a few weeks, your adrenal glands decrease cortisol production. A gradual reduction in prednisone dosage gives your adrenal glands time to resume their normal function but if you stop or taper to quickly severe fatigue, weakness, joint pain and body aches are the usual result.

I know, I know, you are probably shaking your head saying that is exactly how I felt before prednisone! It is so difficult to differentiate these withdrawal symptoms with the symptoms of numerous diseases. The weaning process was about 6 months for Jack and each of these side effects were also the exact symptoms he suffered with Sarcoidosis, fatigue and joint pain being the worst. When I asked if he had any problems with weaning off he said no, but who could really say for sure given the side effects of tapering to quickly mimic the symptoms? This is the, oh so frustrating part about mixing dis-ease and medication. The medication is meant to mask the symptoms but often times only multiplies them with side effects. The good thing is that many of the healing nutrients we talk about in the next few chapters also support proper adrenal function.

After a few months of tapering Jack started his 30 day cleanse, using CleanSMART, which required him to go strictly vegan for a month, drink a minimum of 1 gallon of water every day, no coffee, soda, sugars etc. Then after the cleanse, he tried many different supplements, antioxidant formulas, diets, massages, and essential oils over the course of 3 to 4 months but did not experience much improvement in energy, stamina or pain relief. So his next stab at healing led him to a local yet internationally recognized Doctor of Oriental Medicine (DOM) Laurel Sander who specializes in body work, energy healing, acupuncture, cleansing and more.

During this entire time, Jack continued to ride his bike 2-3 times a week, eat healthy, avoiding all dairy, processed foods and refined sugars. He saw Laurel every three weeks and had treatments which included deep tissue massage, lymphatic massage and acupuncture for 3 months. He would bring home bags of Chinese remedies, supplements, herbs, and tinctures and he faithfully took them all. I remember him drinking the Chinese tinctures; as the stench permeated the kitchen he would plug his nose and chug them down then drink a huge glass of water to rid the rancid taste. He was going to get healthy no matter how or what! Well, maybe not. Even though he did start to experience more energy and less pain his lymph nodes did not change in size or feel so Laurel naturally encouraged him to start high colonic therapy.

Now I am neither for nor against this treatment. High colonic therapy has been effectively used for centuries and we share this option with you because you may want to consider it, especially if you have an impacted colon but please be sure to go to a professional who knows what they are doing. I certainly see the benefits of cleansing the colon and know that it can be very effective in literally removing pounds of decaying matter from the body to improve intestinal immunity, digestion, relieve inflammation, restore regularity and increase the efficiency of the body's natural healing abilities, but Jack was not open to this therapy. Thus came the next chapter in Jack's holistic healing journey which we will talk about in a minute.

Not to break away from the story but are you beginning to see the parallel in allopathic and holistic healing? They both start with a list of maladies that are whittled down through numerous trial and error methods which often lead us back to where we started, that is, until we find the underlying cause. Therein lies the major difference, which is an extremely important one to note. The allopathic philosophy sets out to diagnose and prescribe with medication formulated to mask symptoms so you think you are getting better. These synthetic compounds cause numerous dangerous side effects with extreme physical and financial costs; making the pharmaceutical giants the wealthiest of all. While the holistic philosophy is to find the underlying cause of the symptoms and treat the body entirely by improving your life (even if you can't physically "feel" it) until all ailments are gone without negative side effects or extreme costs. Which one would you prefer?

Most, no actually all of the methods we talk about in this book are referred to in Western medicine as Complementary and Alternative Medicine, better known as CAM. Meaning they can be used to complement (in conjunction with) allopathic treatment or as an alternative to allopathic treatment. You may be wondering how long you have to follow a "regimen" if you will before results. Many people ask us this and to us this has become our lifestyle but for someone just starting I encourage them to give anything they do a minimum of 90 days BEFORE they even consider if it is working or not. Our body depends on the nutrients we feed it to survive, regenerate and replicate on a cellular level. Every 90 to 120 days our bone, skin and blood completely regenerate, so it is important to give any new method a minimum of 90 days to really "feel" if it is making a difference.

Our Body Has A Two-Step Regeneration Process:

1. Eliminate Old Cell Matter - Old matter is transported, via the bloodstream, to the intestines for elimination with food waste.

2. Create/Grow/Regenerate New Cell Matter - New matter is created from nutrients, vitamins, minerals, and protein in food in the intestinal tract. They are absorbed through the intestinal wall into the bloodstream where they are

distributed throughout the body and used as needed, according to the body regeneration schedule.

- ✓ **5 Days - NEW Stomach Lining**
- ✓ **30 Days - NEW Hair - NEW Skin**
- ✓ **45 Days - NEW Liver - NEW DNA Cellular Material**
- ✓ **49 Days - NEW Bladder**
- ✓ **60 Days - NEW Brain Cells, Tissue**
- ✓ **90 Days - NEW Skeleton**
- ✓ **120 Days - NEW Red Blood Cells**

Another thing that commonly interferes with detecting results when making lifestyle changes is medication. Even though many people on prescription medications also make dietary changes, supplement, exercise, hydrate, de-stress, etc. the side effects of the medication will often complicate possible benefits of these changes. For example: Weight gain is one of the most common side effects of corticosteroid use. Even though Jack rode his bike and followed a low carb, high fiber healthy diet he could not lose weight while on prednisone. I think the goal for most is to eventually get off of all medications but the more one is on the more difficult it is to get free.

Ok, back to the story. Jack did not want to experience a high colonic and the cost of the treatments were always a huge stress for us so he decided to finish the supplements and tinctures but search for another possible method for healing. It is wonderful how the universe answers when you ask.

During the summer of 2008, a friend stopped by Calderas, our family restaurant, where I, Dani, lived...just kidding, kind of. He wanted to drop off a bottle of a liquid antioxidant for Jack to try. I remember the day clearly and will forever be grateful to Greg for his courage and perseverance. But by that time, we were on our 5th year battle with Sarcoidosis and I was feeling like there was no hope. I had come to the conclusion that Jack would be wrestling with Sarcoidosis forever and after joining several conversations in different forums I started to fear that it may win! I had decided that as much improvement as Jack experienced over the past 10+ months was as good as he was going to get. Yet Greg had hope. He knew we were trying natural methods and thought maybe this particular supplement would help. The world of supplements is full of antioxidant options. Jack had tried several and I in my mind this was just another one to cross off the list. Besides, we were totally strapped for cash and could not afford to add another supplement. Greg insisted on giving us this one bottle and I graciously accepted. Yet as I thanked him, I was convinced it would be another failure and to be completely honest, at that time I did not know if I could handle more disappointment.

Thank goodness Jack had not reached this negative and hopeless outlook. When I brought the bottle home he looked at the ingredients and said "It's just food, it can't hurt." He started taking an ounce a day and stopped all the other supplements, Chinese tinctures and treatments he was previously trying. We could not afford to do both and if it was going to work, he wanted to know exactly what was working.

Jack: I took one ounce a day for about four months and it did seem to be working. I had more energy and less pain. To my surprise, my lymph started to soften but by the 6th month my results seemed to have plateaued. So, as we most often do, I thought "more was better" and started taking 3-4 ounces a day. It seemed to make me even more tired and in a mental fog. Dani thought I was overdosing on it and started to research other antioxidants and natural anti-inflammatory nutrients.

After Jack's lymph nodes started softening I had a renewed sense of hope. After all, we were told that even if his Sarcoidosis burned out his lymph would not change because they had become fibrocystic. This miraculous change was exactly what my spirit needed to get back in the game! I started researching and found two other supplements that looked promising: Fucoydon and Spectramaxx. Ironically, and not to my excitement, these were also made by a network marketing company but what do you do? He needed something that could help his body arrest the damage of Sarcoidosis and this could be it. We drove 10 hours to the manufacturing facility to see for ourselves how they were formulated and in May 2009, Jack started taking a ½ ounce (15ml) of each daily. He continued to ride his bike, get massages every couple months, and ate a diet high in raw fruits, veggies, void of dairy, soy, processed foods and food additives (we did the best we could).

His overall health continued to improve so by August 2009, he added a third supplement called Eternity and by October

2009 his lymph nodes under his chin were completely back to normal! He had no visible granulomas and no symptoms of Sarcoidosis. He was no longer tired, aching, coughing or dizzy. His lymph nodes were soft and small and he felt like he had his life back! In his words, "I feel like I am 19 again!"

FYI: To this day, Jack still takes ½ ounce of Fucoydon every morning and has continued to do so for the last four plus years. As I stated earlier, this is a lifestyle. In the next chapters, we will study the active ingredients in these supplements & others so you will understand why our entire family supplements and you can add them to your daily regimen, if you so choose.

As much as Jack's improvement shocked us both, it really inspired me! I was curious and had so many questions. I wanted to understand why one supplement would work when so many others did not. What was the secret ingredient or was it a combination of powerful antioxidants? Maybe it was the potency? Why did antioxidants help his body heal? What other health benefits may these nutrients have? Could diet and supplementing help people with other inflammatory diseases? How is it that the lymph nodes started to recede back to their normal size? This was the big question. After all, we were told this was not possible. Could the scar tissue in his lungs eventually repair, too? Everything that had seemed impossible suddenly became possible and my obsession/passion/mission ignited.

Chapter 6: The Missing Link - Permission to Think Outside the Prescription

During this time, I was witness to an influx of customers at Calderas who would inform me of their gluten, lactose, seafood, peanut intolerances and then ask what they could eat on our menu. Yikes! It is like telling the captain of the boat that you do not know how to swim! I should let you know that Calderas is my Mother's creation and just like home, everything is made from scratch. We serve organic meat and heirloom organic produce from the garden, use real and raw ingredients and as I always say, "We make REAL food for real people."

I saw this flood of people with multiple food allergies as a huge neon sign that read, "Houston we've got problems!" I started to engage more with people, asking them how long they had the allergies, if they had any disorders, ailments etc. I was astounded at the epidemic of illnesses people of all ages were experiencing and I wanted to do more than serve them excellent food. I wanted to be a part of educating people, so they could make better, more informed decisions for their health and wellness, too, especially those with Sarcoidosis.

My curiosity got the best of me. I immersed myself in researching everything I could about oxidative stress, reactive oxygen and nitrogen species (ROS and RNS meaning?), fucoidan, sarcoidosis, autoimmune disease, inflammatory response, telomeres, etc. I decided to get on pubmed.gov and the New England Journal of Mediciane to see if there may be any clinical studies connecting Sarcoidosis to oxidative stress. PubMed is the official site for the US National Library of Medicine National Institutes of Health, where medical studies are published for review. I did hundreds upon hundreds of searches and nothing seemed to fit. It was like trying to find a needle in a haystack that may shine some ray of light. FINALLY, I typed in "Sarcoidosis oxidative stress" and whalah -- 120+ studies came up. Jackpot!

After reading through all the medical jargon and doing my best to make sense of it, I found 29 studies linking oxidative stress to the underlying pathology (cause) of sarcoidosis! As I traveled further down the rabbit hole, additional studies revealed that people with sarcoidosis have shorter telomeres than those without Sarc.[4] Many studies suggested that tumor necrosis factor-alpha (TNF-α) plays a major role in the inflammatory process seen in sarcoidosis and other interstitial lung diseases.[5] I will not get too technical but this was all further confirmation of the importance of making these healthy lifestyle changes.

Even though Jack was having such great results, so many people questioned him and his reason for refusing treatment. In a strange way, this confirmation from published medical studies was the permission I needed to continue to think outside the prescription. A small seed of doubt can ruin anything. We had actually made the right choice! What a sigh of relief.

I know I am a geek but I felt like I had found the missing link that held all the pieces together! It was like I had the key to the Holy Grail or something! I was so excited, yet at the same time, dismayed to find this info because in all Jack's years of treatment, never once did a doctor ask how his diet was, if he exercised, or what he did to relieve stress. Never once did they suggest any healthy lifestyle changes to complement his treatment. Never once did anyone talk about eating more raw fruits and veggies or taking supplements in conjunction with treatment. Why not? Did the doctors even know about these studies? This frustration fueled my desire to make this new found knowledge available to everyone with sarcoidosis or with any chronic disease, as well as doctors, too, for that matter.

I started a blog to share my findings with the world. To my surprise, Sarkies from around the globe reached out and I realized we were NOT alone. It was an awakening of ginormous proportions. I would spend my mornings connecting with people via phone, skype or email, then rush off to the restaurant. As I shared what we were doing people were starting to have positive results with so many different diseases: sarcoidosis, diabetes, cancers, psoriasis, chronic fatigue syndrome, referred to as ME in other countries, lupus, migraines etc. I spent so many hours researching, supporting and writing, that one day my youngest said to me, "Mom, you spend more time on the computer than you do with us." OUCH, that stung, but only because it was completely honest, out of love and the absolute truth. This comment smacked me square in the face, so much that I felt the sting in my gut!

I had my own soul searching to do. I had accidentally stumbled into a realm where the world was one. The internet brought my message of hope to life and I could not just shut it off. I was managing our family restaurant, coming home to answer emails, sharing more of my findings online, building an international business through network marketing, and completely missing out on my family. The most important thing in my life, the reason I had quit my job at UPS, the reason I worked so hard in the first place...everything had come full circle for me and now I had to find harmony in life.

I do not like the word 'balance' because I do not feel like we ever achieve it. But harmony, living in the unforced rhythms of grace, that is a beautiful life and there are moments where I actually experience it.☺ I quickly realized I am finite! I can only be in one place at one time, giving my all to one person at a time and in a finite life, time is not our friend. However, that energy I give is infinite. It passes from one to another and helps the world become a better, healthier place and that in turn comes back to my family.

Was it about taking care of us or helping the masses? I was in this strange place where my reach had expanded so rapidly that I soon found myself in a position to host a radio show on Wellness and really get our message of hope out to the world. I was caught between time with my family, raising my children and instilling into them a desire to help mankind or helping mankind myself. Was it possible to lead by example and do both!? Of course it was.

Life is a team sport! So with Jack's and the boys' support, I jumped at the opportunity to host a radio show! Because I am a master of nothing, I called it, "Come learn with me." It was my own selfish way to continue researching and finding solutions, expanding my own knowledge and sharing with the world. I got to interview experts far and wide: neurological chiropractors, functional medicine doctors, integrative medicine doctors, disease survivors, immunologists, chiropractors, and naturopaths. Every show expanded my horizons. The show was such a success that it eventually morphed into "The Medical Insiders" which I co-hosted with naturopathic physician Dr. Richard Powell. We just had one stipulation with our guests; you had to have your own personal story of overcoming "incurable" odds. It was a fabulous way for us to give everyone permission to think outside the prescription and start being their own wellness advocate.

Unfortunately, or maybe fortunately, the comment my youngest son had so poignantly made kept going through my head and after a year I had to re-prioritize. I chose my family and world of friends over the show. It was the absolute best decision but I still miss it. I learned more about wellness in one year than I had in my entire life and the best of the best interviews are now yours to learn from as well!

The shows have been off the air for over a year but I have been editing them to go with this book and I am learning all over again. Our very first show starred Sarcoidosis survivor Jack Walker! (Listen to "Surviving Sarcoidosis" audio).

Nobody knows this but when that show started I was so nervous I could barely breathe, let alone talk. A couple minutes into the show, Jack came sneaking in to let me know that no one could hear me! I panicked, but thanks to him I made it through the first show and swore my first show would be my last. LOL! My hope is our lecture at OHSU this fall goes much better than my first radio show! Needless to say, I was on air every Wednesday at 10:00 am for the next 52 weeks. Sometimes in life we are challenged to do something completely outside our box and most of the time we survive and grow more than we could ever have imagined.

I would often say on the show that, "Wellness is the connection of paths between knowledge and action." As you read this book and listen to the audios, I can only hope that you spread the knowledge, but most importantly, implement it into your own life; after all education beats medication...right? Wink, wink.

In the next chapters we do our best to cover a ton of information on nutrients that fight inflammation, support lung function, repair organ and tissue damage, etc. You will find the resources and recipes in Chapter 12 very helpful. You will gain a great understanding of the power your body has to heal itself when given the proper nutrients, as well as, alternative methods for detecting and preventing disease before it starts. The audios are filled with pearls of wisdom from leading health experts in their respective fields. You are literally getting a free consultation with 10 different specialists!

I am kind of jumping ahead in our story here, but I have to tell you about a non-invasive scan that costs 1/10th what a PET or CT scan costs and is just as effective (possibly more effective) in detecting inflammation, tumors, etc. years before these traditional methods. Have you ever heard of Thermography?

One of our guests was thermographer Jeanie Nelson, from Medical Thermography Northwest. A friend of mine called me one day about a lump she found in her breast and asked me if I had ever heard of thermography. I said, "No, what is it?" That was when my wellness world expanded yet again.

When I found out that Thermography was a non-invasive thermal scan to detect inflammation within the body, I was all over it. I immediately called Jeannie and asked her to be a guest on the show. Jack and I booked our Thermography scans during a time when she was going to be near us and the rest is history.

You see, after I quit my job at UPS, Jack could no longer get health "sickness" insurance. I would call companies and as soon as I said the word "Sarcoidosis" they would say "Sorry but we do not write policies for that," and the conversation was over. Jack would have to wait for five years (which we did) before an insurance company would even consider him. We were not willing to spend $3,000-$5,000 on a CT scan to confirm that his granulomas were indeed gone. We could no longer see the swollen tumors under his chin so we just took it at "face" value that he was in remission – pun intended.☺ But we were always curious and did not know of any alternatives. The cost of a CT scan was one hurdle and radiation was another. We were doing our best to stay away from health hazards and it just did not make sense to willingly expose him to radiation through CT scan.

In May 2012, almost three years to the day since we considered Jack in remission that he had Thermography. His results showed some inflammation in his gums, confirming that he was well overdue for a cleaning. There was also some residual inflammation in his lymph nodes under his chin but it was minimal and could be taken care of with a more stringent alkaline diet. The most amazing thing was that there was no inflammation in the lungs or mediastinum! The test did not detect any tumors, growths, or granulomas anywhere and that was confirmation enough that his Sarcoidosis was in remission for sure! YAHOOOO.

The scan for Jack was only $295.00! This was less than we owed for Jack's initial CT scan, eight years prior, *after* the insurance paid 80%! It just goes to show that alternatives can be much less costly than main stream medicine and usually much safer, too. If we would have known about thermography before Jack was diagnosed, we would have certainly used this alternative to invasive scans for detecting any changes in tumors throughout his treatment. Thermography is well-known mostly for early detection of breast cancer but it can be used for early detection of any inflammatory disease.

In the case of diabetes, for example, Jeannie showed me a picture of someone's hands. They were completely red (hot and inflamed) which she said is a tell-tale sign of diabetes. This is the beauty of Thermography; it is inexpensive and extremely effective in detecting the beginning signs of a disease so lifestyle changes can be made early on to prevent the dis-ease completely. The picture below states that after 2 years of development a tumor only has 256 cells in it and is already detectable by thermography but by the time the tumor is large enough to be detected by mammography it has almost 270 million cells and has been developing for 7 years! Given this information I think it smart to get regular thermographs every 24-36 months.

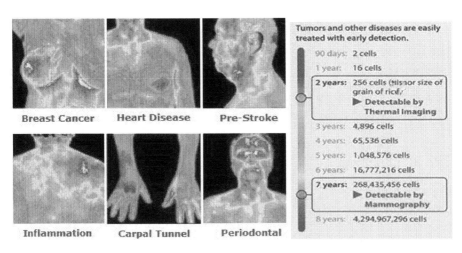

Breast Cancer   Heart Disease   Pre-Stroke

Inflammation   Carpal Tunnel   Periodontal

Tumors and other diseases are easily treated with early detection.

90 days: 2 cells

1 year: 16 cells

2 years: 256 cells (sussaor size of grain of rice/
▶ Detectable by Thermal Imaging

3 years: 4,896 cells

4 years: 65,536 cells

5 years: 1,048,576 cells

6 years: 16,777,216 cells

7 years: 268,435,456 cells
▶ Detectable by Mammography

8 years: 4,294,967,296 cells

Chapter 6 Trivia: What is Thermography? (listen to "What Is Thermography" audio)

Thermography is a non-invasive, non-contact tool that uses the heat from your body to aid in making diagnosis of a host of health care conditions. Thermography is completely safe and uses no radiation.

Digital Infrared Thermal Imaging is a unique technology that takes a picture and creates a map of the infrared patterns of the body. It is different than other screening tools because it helps us to see function (physiology). MRI and X-ray detect anatomical changes; however, they miss such things as active inflammation or angiogenesis (increased blood supply as found in cancer).

Thermography was approved by the FDA for breast cancer screening in 1982. It can detect early danger signs in the body years before other tools. It has been shown to be effective in finding early signs of breast cancer up to eight years before the mammogram.

There are three areas when Thermography is useful:
1. Inflammatory Phenomena - This could include early detection of cardiovascular disease, arthritis, fibromyalgia or trauma such as strains, sprains or chronic pain.
2. Neovascular Phenomena - Cancer is fed by the body's own blood supply. This development of early vascularity is detected well before anatomical

changes occur that would be detected with other screening tools.

3. Neurological Phenomena – In Chronic Regional Pain Syndrome, nerve irritation can cause referred pain in other areas. Circulatory deficits are easily seen in thermographic images.

A full body screening covers all regions of the body with no less than 28 images. A region of interest can be used for focalized screening, such as breast screening, thyroid, lymph, heart, etc.

Thermography has been comprehensively researched for over 30 years. While it is not a replacement for mammography, it may have many valuable assets, including early detection of neovascular (blood supply) patterns, adjunct to inconclusive mammograms, improved detection for women with dense breasts or implants, or a reasonable alternative for women who refuse mammogram. Below is a sample of over 800 studies in the index-medicus. They represent some important findings and value of thermography.

Fast facts:
- In 1982, the FDA approved breast thermography as an adjunct diagnostic breast cancer screening procedure.
- Of the extensive research conducted since the late 1950's, well over 300,000 women have been included as study participants.
- The size of the studies are very large: 10,000, 37,000, 60,000, 85,000.

- Some studies have followed participants up to 12 years.
- Strict standardized interpretation protocols have been established for 15 years to remedy problems with early research.
- Breast thermography has an average sensitivity and specificity of 90%.
- An abnormal thermogram is 10 times more significant as a future risk indicator for breast cancer than a first order family history.
- A persistent abnormal thermogram carries with it a 22 times higher risk of future breast cancer.
- Extensive clinical trials have shown that breast thermography significantly augments the long term survival rates of its recipients by as much as 61%. When used as a multimodal approach (clinical exam plus mammography plus thermography), 95% of early stage cancers will be detected.

Thermography is being used in sports medicine, dentistry, podiatry, chiropractic, orthopedics rheumatology, and neurology, in a variety of support or adjunctive diagnostic roles. It was soon realized that thermography could clearly, objectively, and easily demonstrate the physiological component of pain and injury, especially to the spinal column, due to car accidents, job injuries, and a host of other "tort" related law suits. Everyone involved has benefited from these positive test findings, which could be clearly shown to a jury. Everyone, that is, except the defendant insurance industry.

Needless to say, the insurance industry in the United States placed an all-out effort to diminish the value of thermography in courts of law due to high litigation costs. Eventually, lobbying efforts at the American Medical Association's (AMA) House of Delegates and at Medicare, brought about the removal of thermography coverage by most insurance companies and greatly reduced the utilization of thermography in the United States. This was most unfortunate for the patients who could clearly benefit from thermal imaging.

Is it accurate? Yes, as a routine screening tool, it has been shown to be 97% effective at detecting benign vs. malignant breast abnormalities. Another study tracked 1537 women with abnormal thermo grams for 12 years. They had normal mammograms and physical exams. Within five years, 40% of the women developed malignancies. The researchers commented, "an abnormal thermogram is the single most important marker of high risk for the future development of breast cancer." These results have been repeated over and over again for nearly 30 years.

Is It safe? While a variety of studies have called into question the safety of cumulative exposures to radiation, this is not the case with thermography. Thermography emits nothing, it only takes an image. Nothing touches you and it is quick and painless. This all makes thermography great for frequent screening with no chance of danger. Even pregnant and nursing mothers can benefit. It is non-invasive, does not use radiation, does not compress the breast and poses absolutely no harm to the woman whatsoever.

Is Thermal imaging different from mammography or ultrasound? Yes. Unlike mammography and ultrasound, Digital Infrared Thermal Imaging (DITI) is a test of *physiology*. It detects and records the infrared heat radiating from the surface of the body. It can help in early detection and monitoring of abnormal physiology and the establishment of risk factors for the development or existence of cancer.

Mammography and ultrasound are tests of anatomy. They look at structure. When a tumor has grown to a size that is large enough and dense enough to block an x-ray beam (mammography) or sound wave (ultrasound), it produces an image that can be detected by a trained radiologist.

Neither mammogram, ultrasound, nor Thermography (DITI) can diagnose cancer. Only a biopsy can diagnose cancer. However, when DITI, mammograms, ultrasounds, and clinical exams are used together, the best possible evaluation of breast health can be made.

Chapter 7: Oxidative Stress, Sarcoidosis, ILDs and 60+ Diseases

"The amount of antioxidants that you maintain in your body is directly related to how long you will live."– Richard G. Cutler, MD

I know I got off track sharing Thermography with you but what a wonderful detection tool to prevent disease from occurring! As Jack continued to improve I continued to research. Once I finally found the studies that confirmed we were on the right track, I was ready to take Sarcoidosis head on. Live, unedited and on air!

Before we talk more about the studies I found years ago, let me share with you a very recent published work from this year (2013) about Sarcoidosis, entitled; A Review of Current and Emerging Pharmacological Treatments for Sarcoidosis:

> "Sarcoidosis is a multisystem granulomatous disease of unknown cause. The disease most commonly affects the lung, but any organ can be involved. Sarcoidosis has a variable natural course from an asymptomatic state to a progressive disease, that, on occasion, may be life threatening. Treatment decisions concerning sarcoidosis are problematic for many reasons. First, treatment is often associated with significant side effects. Therefore, treatment may cause more harm than the disease, especially since sarcoidosis may never cause significant symptoms. Second, although sarcoidosis is often well

controlled with corticosteroids, many corticosteroid side effects result from chronic use.

Therefore, even when sarcoidosis is well controlled with corticosteroids, corticosteroid-sparing medications may be required over time. Third, the treatment of sarcoidosis varies, to some degree, depending on the organ or organs that may be involved. Fourth, because sarcoidosis is not a common disease, minimal evidence-based data exist on which to support treatment decisions.

Corticosteroid therapy is considered first line therapy for acute and chronic sarcoidosis in which a decision is made to treat. Despite the nearly universal opinion that corticosteroids are the drug of choice for almost all forms of sarcoidosis, no pharmacologic treatments for sarcoidosis have been approved by the US Food and Drug Administration. Corticosteroids act mainly by repression of inflammatory genes including interferon-gamma (IFN-γ) and tumor necrosis factor (TNF)-alpha that are important cytokines in the development of the sarcoid granuloma. A number of additional inflammatory cytokines that are involved in granuloma formation and maintenance are responsive to the anti-inflammatory properties of corticosteroids.

There is no prospective data to guide the dose, duration, or tapering of corticosteroids in sarcoidosis. Guiding principles are offered in the official sarcoidosis consensus statement of the American Thoracic Society (ATS)/European Respiratory Society (ERS)/World Association of Sarcoidosis and Other Granulomatous Diseases (WASOG)."[6]

Now excuse me but the name of the study is, A Review of Current and Emerging Pharmacological Treatments for Sarcoidosis, so where the heck is the information on the EMERGING treatments? Apparently nothing has changed, they just reiterating the last 50+ years of treating Sarcoid. How frustrating!!!

We all want a cure so badly but the last 5 years of researching I've begun to believe that only 1 million people with a disease is NOT enough for pharmaceutical companies to 'pay' attention. In other words, there's no money in developing medications or performing studies for such a small population. But, the study does give us a few breadcrumbs. The sentence: Corticosteroids act mainly by repression of inflammatory genes including interferon-gamma (IFN-γ) and tumor necrosis factor (TNF)-alpha that are important cytokines in the development of the sarcoid granuloma. This sentence gives me some direction. If I had not already researched natural TNF-a and IFN-y inhibitors, I would have after reading this study. ☺

Now that we all have a better idea of when Dr consider treating Sarcoidosis and the main reason why corticosteroids are the treatment of choice, let us first talk about oxidative stress. In the next chapter we will study some nutrients found in nature that have been clinically proven to inhibit interferon-gamma (IFN-γ) and tumor necrosis factor (TNF)-alpha just as corticosteroids do! These nutrients also fight oxidative stress. As Carl C. Pfeiffer, M.D., Ph.D. said, "For every drug that benefits a patient, there is a natural substance that can achieve the same effect." — Pfeiffer's Law.

Below are five of the 29+ plus published scientific studies suggesting that a diet high in broad spectrum antioxidant nutrition could help slow and/or reverse the signs of Sarcoidosis. I have not based all of my hypotheses on these studies but they certainly were confirmation of our choices. I have summarized the findings but these studies can be researched by going to www.pubmed.gov and typing "sarcoidosis oxidative stress" in the search bar! If you have a different disease you can do the same to find out if it too is related to oxidative stress.

First of all oxidative stress is an imbalance between oxidants: reactive oxygen species (ROS) and reactive nitrogen species (RNS) and antioxidants that may affect lipids, DNA, carbohydrates and proteins. Science has identified around 2200 different groups of free radicals (oxidants). According to these studies, Sarcoidosis patients have much higher oxidative stress levels than people without Sarcoid and according to the book *Oxidative Stress, Inflammation, and Health,* a technical guide to Oxidative stress and disease, oxidative stress is linked to more than 60 diseases including cancer, allergies, heart disease, diabetes, rheumatoid arthritis, lupus, asthma, Alzheimer's and many more.

Study 1. ROS are responsible for the tissue damage in interstitial lung diseases (ILDs) such as lung fibrosis or sarcoidosis. This is a lead in the development of new therapies and of <u>suggesting optimal antioxidant dietary regimes</u>.[7]

Study 2. A potential role of oxidative stress in the step-by-step development of a disease and the chain of events leading to diffuse lung diseases (DLD) has been demonstrated. Increased oxidant levels and decreased antioxidant defenses can contribute to the progression of idiopathic pulmonary fibrosis, sarcoidosis, pneumoconiosis and pulmonary fibrosis associated with systemic sclerosis.[8]

Study 3. Future studies should explore the clinical relevance of the relation of oxidative stress, antioxidant therapy and cardiac dysfunction in sarcoidosis.[9]

Study 4. <u>Sarcoidosis patients might benefit from antioxidant supplementation</u> not only by empowering the relatively low protection against ROS but also by reducing inflammation.[10] Re-read this one once more!

Study 5. Oxidative mechanisms are currently discussed as playing a crucial role in the pathogenesis of inflammatory lung diseases. Oxidative stress increases in sarcoidosis might be due to both increase in lipid peroxidation and decrease in antioxidant status (PON1).[11]

These five studies all confirm that a diet high in raw fruits and vegetables (excellent sources for antioxidants) and/or supplementing your diet with antioxidants can benefit people with sarcoidosis. Even though a these studies suggest that Dr recommend dietary change and give direction into future studies, neither seems to be taking place.

It is our goal to bring awareness to these options so we can all be informed and empowered to take back our health rather than feeling lost, alone and hopeless. As I said earlier, I went through frustration, anger, etc. that we were never informed of any of this. I had to harness my anger. I chose to believe that doctors themselves are not aware of these studies. I have since had confirmation that much of this information is not translating into practice. Yet, that is. It is Jack's and my goal to help make that happen! ☺ ☺ ☺

When we speak at the Sarcoidosis Conference at OHSU this fall, we will share these findings, testimonies from Sarkies, and present our case before Sarcoidosis specialists in hope that they will embrace and more importantly incorporate these findings into treatment options. Coming closer to an integrative medicine approach, much like Cancer Treatment Centers of America have would be wonderful. We encourage you to share this book with your specialists, too.

So what is oxidative stress? It takes a long time for cells to mutate but this is exactly what happens after years of oxidative stress caused by free radical damage. To understand oxidative stress we must first know what a free radical is. A free radical is an unstable oxygen molecule that must find another electron to make itself complete. In order to do this, the free radical begins randomly

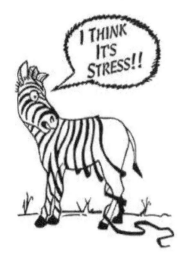

bombarding your cells, resulting in injury to the surrounding cell tissue and causing oxidative stress. Free radicals steal electrons from healthy cells and turn them into free radicals as well. Antioxidants stop free radical damage by donating an electron without becoming a damaging free radical.

In other words, free radicals are the little ghosts on Pacman that kill him, only worse; when a free radical (ghost) attacks a cell (Pacman) it turns that cell into another free radical (ghost) and then those two free radicals turn two more cells into free radicals and those four turn four more. You get the picture. As we get older the level of free radical build up in the body increases. The good news is our bodies naturally produce antioxidants. But

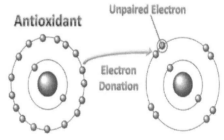

the bad news is many free radicals in our environment are synthetic and made of a chemistry that our body's natural antioxidants (SOD, catalase and glutathione) cannot interact with to neutralize. We must get these additional antioxidants from food or supplement sources. Due to the lack of proper nutrition, toxic environments and moderate exercise, the number of free radicals in our bodies vastly outnumber the number of antioxidants. This oxidative stress leads to premature aging and chronic disease.

You can start fighting free radicals by adding more raw foods into your daily diet. We drink green smoothies. It is a great way to get 4-6 servings of fresh fruits and veggies as well as "hide" all the healthy stuff so the kids get their veggies, too. We share several yummy recipes in Chapter 12.

Signs and Symptoms of Oxidative Stress

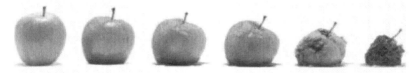

These apples demonstrate how oxidative stress breaks down your cells, causing premature aging and disease.

1. A manageable headache, indigestion, constipation, rash, sore joint and muscles. Your body is trying to tell you something.

2. A decrease in blood levels of micro-nutrients and trace elements, as well as, many vitamins. As the cells are damaged by free radicals they are not able to assimilate nutrients as well thus causing further damage.

3. Inflammation seems to be at the base of oxidative stress. As cells mutate our immune system is overworked and eventually inflammation sets in. Inflammation is our bodies' natural and appropriate response of the immune system (your body's defense system) to infection and trauma, but hidden inflammation that runs amok is at the root of all chronic illnesses, including conditions like sarcoidosis, heart disease, obesity, diabetes, dementia, depression, cancer, IBS and even autism.

4. Metabolic syndrome is the generic name of chronic conditions such as obesity, hypertension, diabetes mellitus, and hyperlipidemia. All of these conditions are the result of inactivity, poor nutrition and oxidative stress but remember, every one of them start with a "manageable" symptom before they become debilitating diseases.

Health Benefits Of Antioxidants
Science has linked more than 60 diseases to oxidative stress caused by free radical damage. Antioxidants fight this free radical damage and boost your body's natural ability to stay healthy.

Central Nervous System
- Many antioxidants cross the blood brain barrier to help protect the brain from free radical damage, thereby helping the brain remain healthy.
- Protect against dementia, Alzheimer's disease, Parkinson's disease, and stroke.

Liver

- Boost liver detoxification function, helping to eliminate toxins and carcinogens.

Heart

- Help to prevent and reverse heart disease.
- Lower your risk of developing (and dying from) coronary heart disease.
- Indirectly helps to lower blood pressure.
- May raise HDL, "good cholesterol", and lower LDL, "bad cholesterol", thereby decreasing risk of developing heart disease.
- Help prevent the oxidation of LDL, thereby decreasing cholesterol deposits from forming (atherosclerosis).

Lung

- Help to alleviate lung disorders, including asthma, cigarette smoke-induced injury, and emphysema/COPD.

Circulation

- Relax blood vessels, thereby improving blood circulation and helping to normalize blood pressure.
- Help to decrease blood viscosity (keep blood cells slippery) and prevent thrombus formation (blood clots from forming), thereby helping to prevent heart attacks and strokes.
- Strengthen blood vessel walls and decrease the risk of bleeding.
- Increase nitric oxide levels. Nitric oxide has positive effects on blood vessels, prevents inflammation, helps to lower blood pressure, and improves blood flow to the heart, lungs, kidneys, and brain.

Immune System

- Boost immune function and protect against many types of infections.
- Have antiviral, antibacterial, antihistamine, and even anti-cancer properties.
- Inhibit the enzyme necessary for histamine production (antihistamine effect), thereby alleviating hay fever, allergy symptoms, eczema, and asthma.
- Generally shown to dramatically reduce the likelihood of many cancers; also, slows the progression of existing cancers.

Skin

- Help keep skin smooth, flexible, and more youthful.
- Reduce wrinkles, sun spots, and decrease risk of skin cancer.
- Strengthen and repair connective tissue and inhibit the body's enzymes that break down collagen, thereby protecting the skin from age-related injury.
- Help alleviate skin disorders, including sunburn (UV/solar inflammation), general burns, psoriasis, eczema, and allergic skin conditions.

Eyes

- Protect against visual loss that occurs with aging, i.e., diabetic retinopathy, macular degeneration, cataracts, and degenerative retinal damage (age-related).

There are literally thousands of high antioxidant foods but here are a few to eat more of: small red beans, blueberries, cranberries, blackberries, dried prunes, red delicious apples, granny smith apples, pecans, sweet cherries, black plums, kale, spinach, brocili, dark chocolate (oh yeah!) and so many more but remember they must be organic and raw is best! It is important to note that a high dose of Vitamin C is NOT sufficient – as there are over 2200 groups of free radicals and Vitamin C only combats a few of these groups. We all need a broad spectrum of fruits and vegetables to receive the many health benefits of antioxidants. The basis is simple; just as Hippocrates said in 450 B.C., "Food is thy medicine." In today's world we need to say, "REAL food is thy medicine."

On top of fighting oxidative stress we want to eat foods that inhibit tumor necrosis factor-alpha (TNF-α). Studies have found that TNF-α, a 17.5-kd protein, plays a significant role in antigen-stimulated, cell-mediated immune responses and in the development of noncaseating granulomas in a variety of diseases, including Sarcoidosis. In sarcoidosis high levels of TNF-α released from alveolar macrophages seem to correlate with disease progression.[12] Thus eating a diet high in anti-inflammatory foods which naturally inhibit tumor necrosis factor-alpha (TNF-α), as well as, daily practices that will help your body stop and possibly reverse this disease can be the turning point in your health. Natural TNF-a inhibitors include; fucoidan[13], curcumin (Tumeric)[14], quercetin and resveratrol[15], green tea[16], cat's claw[17], CoQ10[18], and tart cherry juice. If you are suffering from a different disease and would like to know if inhibiting TNF-a would be beneficial you can search the name of your dis-ease and the words tumor necrosis factor alpha but beware, it could lead down a rabbit hole of possibilities that will require you to be your own private investigator or "medical insider" as we referred to in our radio show *The Medical Insiders*.

As we continue to implement what we learn into our own lives we have seen Jack go into complete remission, Trent's allergies improve, and my migraines go from one or two every three months to one a year. As we share these findings with others who choose to implement them into their daily lives, we have witnessed people's A1C drop 2 to 3 points within 30 days, children with psoriasis become rash free within 60 days, several women with chronic fatigue become pain free and regain energy, and many Sarcoid survivors are living a much better quality of life.

I will share one quick story about a friend with brain cancer who was on her 2nd round of chemo treatments and could barely function for a week after each treatment. We gave her a ton of information and studies showing that fucoidan (a natural nutrient found in brown seaweed which we will talk about in detail soon) helped weaken cancer cells so chemotherapy and radiation would be more effective and at the same time strengthen and protect healthy cells from chemotherapy and radiation. Given the information, she decided to start taking a half-ounce of concentrated fucoidan five days before her next chemotherapy and the day after her treatment she was up and able to go grocery shopping and run errands! She was thrilled and three weeks later when she went for her next treatment, her doctor commented on how much her hair was growing back, too!

Chapter 7 Trivia: "Food Stuffs" to Avoid (Listen to *Toxic Food Syndrome* audio)

AVOID: Dairy, high glycemic carbohydrates, processed, canned, boxed foods, red meat (read meat is one of the most acidic and complicated foods for us to digest).

When reading labels here are the top 10 food additives to avoid:

1. Artificial Sweeteners. Aspartame, (E951) more popularly known as Nutrasweet and Equal, is found in foods labeled "diet" or "sugar free." Aspartame is believed to be carcinogenic and accounts for more reports of adverse reactions than all other foods and food additives combined. Aspartame is a neurotoxin and carcinogen. Known to erode intelligence and affect short-term memory, the components of this toxic sweetener may lead to a wide variety of ailments including brain tumor, diseases like lymphoma, diabetes, multiple sclerosis, Parkinson's, Alzheimer's, fibromyalgia, and chronic fatigue, emotional disorders like depression and anxiety attacks, dizziness, headaches, nausea, mental confusion, migraines and seizures. Acesulfame-K, a relatively new artificial sweetener found in baking goods, gum and gelatin, has not been thoroughly tested, but has been linked to kidney tumors. Found in: Diet or sugar free sodas, diet Coke, Coke Zero, Jello (and other gelatins), desserts, sugar free gum, drink mixes, baking goods, table top sweeteners, cereal, breath mints, pudding, Kool-Aid, ice tea, chewable vitamins, and toothpaste.

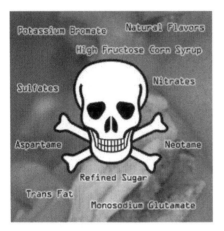

2. High Fructose Corn Syrup. High fructose corn syrup (HFCS) is a highly-refined artificial sweetener (found in almost all processed foods) which has become the number one source of calories in America. HFCS packs on the pounds faster than any other ingredient, increases your LDL ("bad") cholesterol levels, and contributes to the development of diabetes and tissue damage, among other harmful effects. Found in: Most processed foods, breads, candy, flavored yogurts, salad dressings, canned vegetables, and cereals.

3. Monosodium Glutamate (MSG / E621). MSG is an amino acid used as a flavor enhancer in soups, salad dressings, chips, frozen entrees, and many restaurant foods. MSG is known as an excitotoxin, a substance which overexcites cells to the point of damage or death. Studies show that regular consumption of MSG may result in adverse side effects which include depression, disorientation, eye damage, fatigue, headaches, and obesity. MSG affects the neurological pathways of the brain and disengaged the "I am full" function which explains the effects of weight gain. Found in: Chinese food (Chinese Restaurant Syndrome), many snacks, chips, cookies, seasonings, most Campbell Soup products, frozen dinners, and lunch meats.

4. Trans Fat. Trans fats are used to enhance and extend the shelf life of food products and is among the most dangerous substances that you can consume. Trans fats are formed by a process called hydrogenation. Numerous studies show that trans-fat increases LDL cholesterol levels while decreasing HDL ("good") cholesterol, increases the risk of heart attacks, heart disease and strokes, and contributes to increased inflammation, diabetes and other health problems. Oils and fat are now forbidden on the Danish market if they contain trans fatty acids exceeding two per cent, a move that effectively bans partially hydrogenated oils.
Found in: Margarine, chips and crackers, baked goods, and fast foods.

5. Common Food Dyes. Studies show that artificial colorings which are found in soda, fruit juices, and salad dressings, may contribute to behavioral problems in children and lead to a significant reduction in IQ.
Blue #1 and Blue #2 (E133). Banned in Norway, Finland and France. May cause chromosomal damage.
Found in: Candy, cereal, sodas, sports drinks and pet foods.
Red dye # 3 (also Red #40 – a more current dye) (E124). Banned in 1990 after eight years of debate from use in many foods and cosmetics. This dye continues to be on the market until supplies run out! Has been proven to cause thyroid cancer and chromosomal damage in laboratory animals. May also interfere with brain-nerve transmission.
Found in: Fruit cocktail, maraschino cherries, cherry pie mix, ice cream, candy, bakery products and more.
Yellow #6 (E110) and Yellow Tartrazine (E102). Banned in

Norway and Sweden. Increases the number of kidney and adrenal gland tumors in laboratory animals. May cause chromosomal damage.
Found in: American cheese, macaroni and cheese, candy, carbonated beverages, lemonade and more.

6. Sodium Sulfite (E221). Preservative used in wine-making and other processed foods. According to the FDA, approximately one in 100 people is sensitive to sulfites in food. The majority of these individuals are asthmatic, suggesting a link between asthma and sulfites. Individuals who are sulfite sensitive may experience headaches, breathing problems, and rashes. In severe cases, sulfites can actually cause death by closing down the airway altogether, leading to cardiac arrest.
Found in: Wine and dried fruit.

7. Sodium Nitrate/Sodium Nitrite. Sodium Nitrate is used as a preservative, coloring and flavoring in bacon, ham, hot dogs, luncheon meats, corned beef, smoked fish and other processed meats. This ingredient is actually highly carcinogenic once it enters the human digestive system. There it forms a variety of nitrosamine compounds that enter the bloodstream and wreak havoc with a number of internal organs: the liver and pancreas, in particular. Sodium nitrite is widely regarded as a toxic ingredient. The USDA actually tried to ban this additive in the 1970s but was vetoed by food manufacturers who complained they had no alternative for preserving packaged meat products. It is actually a color fixer, and it makes old, dead meats appear fresh and vibrant. This is why we do not buy meat

from the store.
Found in: Hotdogs, bacon, ham, luncheon meat, cured meats, corned beef, smoked fish or any other type of processed meat.

8. Butylated hydroxyanisole (BHA) and butylated hydrozyttoluene (BHT). BHA and BHT (E320) are preservatives found in cereals, chewing gum, potato chips, and vegetable oils. This common preservative keeps foods from changing color, changing flavor or becoming rancid. Effects the neurological system of the brain, alters behavior and has potential to cause cancer. BHA and BHT are oxidants which form cancer-causing reactive compounds in your body.
Found in: Potato chips, gum, cereal, frozen sausages, enriched rice, lard, shortening, candy, and jello.

9. Sulfur Dioxide (E220). Sulfur additives are toxic. In the United States of America, the FDA has prohibited their use on raw fruit and vegetables. Adverse reactions include: bronchial problems, particularly in those prone to asthma, hypotension (low blood pressure), flushing tingling sensations or anaphylactic shock. It also destroys vitamins B1 and E. Not recommended for consumption by children. The International Labour Organization says to avoid E220 if you suffer from conjunctivitis, bronchitis, emphysema, bronchial asthma, or cardiovascular disease.
Found in: Beer, sodas, dried fruit, juices, cordials, wine, vinegar, and potato products.

10. Potassium Bromate. Potassium bromate is an additive used to increase volume in some white flour, breads, and rolls. Potassium bromate is known to cause cancer in animals. Even small amounts in bread can create problems for humans.
Found in: Breads.

Chapter 8: We Are What We Absorb So What Should We Eat?

"You can trace every sickness, every disease and every ailment to a mineral deficiency."
Dr. Linus Pauling

After reading the list of food stuffs to avoid, many people ask, "What can I eat?". Our body is made up of 100 TRILLION cells and each cell generates 100s of chemical reactions every day. Nutrients found in REAL foods nourish every cell with the vitamins, minerals, amino acids, etc., needed to perform these biochemical reactions and keep us healthy. At the chemical level, food is our brain's primary link to its environment and to its evolution. Our diet affects the brain chemicals which influence how we feel and behave. The thought processes and emotional reactions we have every day are completely connected to what we eat. Depending on what you eat...this could be a very scary concept! Especially in today's world of instant meals and soil depletion; to "feel" good we must eat great. Therefore, we need to read labels, stay away from highly processed foods, including excite-toxins, sodas, and dairy, unless it is raw and organic, other than eggs. Why are eggs considered dairy anyway? I never understood that.

We know firsthand the challenge of changing your daily diet. You would laugh or scream if you had to go shopping with my youngest and I. Because of Trent's food sensitivities and our awareness we spend most of our time reading labels. After reading 8 or 9 labels and not putting a single thing in the cart he is ready to explode! Out of frustration he will ask/exclaim "Why does everything have high fructose corn syrup, soy, MSG, aspartame....in it!"

It's really a great question. After all, none of us would ever set out

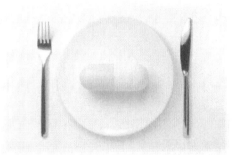

"People are fed by the Food Industry, which pays no attention to health,

and are treated by the Health Industry, which pays no attention to food."

to make a meal for our family with ingredients proven to cause cancer, neurological disorders, respiratory problems, etc but the fact is we buy pre-packaged, boxed meals with these ingredients every day. Food manufacturers are in business to make a profit and if high fructose corn syrup costs half the price of real sugar or MSG makes us eat twice as much...well, regardless of how it affects our health, these ingredients literally make them cents. I try to explain this to my boys every time they come through the door with some goodie they bought.

When we found out Trent could not eat potatoes we started really paying attention to food labels. Little did we know everything has some form of potato byproduct in it. Anything with the word "enriched", yes most breads, pastas, crackers, and it's pretty much a guarantee that he can't eat it. He was only 5 when we finally found out what was going on with him so I explained it like this: (For your information: We have a cat named Batman and a dog named Robbin, yes our kids are very clever.)

I asked Trent, "Would you feed Batman and Robbin stuff that you know would make them sick? Like monster energy drinks, microwaved burritos, corn dogs, French fries, boxed macaroni and cheese, Top Ramen, Oreos and sour patch kids?" He laughed and said, "Mom, they would die." He instantly got it and has been a label reader ever since.

So I will ask you, "How healthy would your pet be if their dish was filled with coffee in the morning, Pepsi for the rest of the day and the food dish rivaled the boxed foods isle at your local grocery store?" We love our pets and many times we take better care of them than we do ourselves. Don't we?!

Having said all this I will get down off my soap box and say that, in every aspect including diet, life is more about what you add than what you take away. Jack and I challenge you to add healthy, nutrient dense foods to your daily diet! Instead of taking anything away, simply start by adding one Green Smoothie to your daily diet. (See recipes in Chapter 12 and Listen to "Powered By Green Smoothies" with Sergei Boutenko)

Jack and I are not nutritionists but the nutrients we've talk about already and the foods below are main staples in our diet. We GO LIVE as much as we can. We choose raw, organic foods, whole grains, avoid diary, processed foods, refined sugars, soy and GMO.

Vegetables and Fruits: Asparagus, Mangoes, Apples, Melons, Apricots, Artichoke, Onions, Arugula, Beets,

Oranges, Broccoli, Parsley and Parsley Root, Peaches, Horseradish (grated), Pears, Cabbage, Pepper, Green and Red Bell Pepper, Plums, Carrots, Lettuce, Cucumbers, Cauliflower, Radishes, Celery, Chards, Rhubarb, Cherries, Chicory , Romaine, Chives, Cilantro, Garlic, Eggplant, Endives, Spinach, Escarole, Avocado, Green Beans, Tangerines, Tomatoes, Grapefruit, Grapes, and Coconut.

Protein: Nuts, Legumes, Eggs (farm fresh or organic), Peanut Butter, Almond Butter, Hemp Seed/Powder, and Chia Seeds. If you are a meat eater go for fish or chicken but only when organic and make them the side dish a couple times a week rather than the main course of every meal. The average 150-pound person needs 55 to 68 grams of protein a day, or about 20 grams of protein per meal. Dairy generally contains about 8 grams per serving, while an ounce of nuts or seeds, or an egg white, boast 6 grams each. A half cup of legumes, such as cooked beans or lentils, contains about 10 grams. Even grains and vegetables generally have a gram or two of protein. Quinoa actually contains 6 grams of protein per serving!

Starch: Squash, Sweet Potatoes, Brown Rice, Quinoa, Whole Oatmeal, Spelt, Potatoes, Yams, Coconut Flour, Arrowroot, and Whole Grain Bread (Dave's Killer Bread is the ONLY one I can find that is actually 100% organic and soy free – and it is excellent, too).

Dried fruit: Peaches, Dates, Figs, Apricots, Prunes, Raisins, Mango, and Apples.

Vinegar (wine, balsamic, cider), Coconut Oil, Flax Oil, Hemp Oil, Olive Oil, and Flax Seed.

Spices: Allspice, Anise, Bay Leaves, Currants, Coriander, Dill, Fennel, Marjoram, Rosemary, Sage, Saffron, Tarragon, Thyme, Sorrel, Summer Savory, Turmeric, and Oregano.

Sugar: If you are going to eat sugar, go with honey. A study in *The Scientific World Journal* found that when people were given equal amounts of either honey or sugar, those in the honey group actually saw a reduction in both weight *and* body fat. Honey has trace amounts of niacin, riboflavin, thiamin, vitamin B6, free-radical fighting antioxidants, and, in raw form, gut-friendly bacteria. It's low glycemic index keeps sugar levels in check and it is up to 50 percent sweeter than the white stuff - so your sweet tooth will be satisfied with less. Maple syrup, molasses, Stevia and xylitol are a few additional options, but honey is at the top of our list.

Salt and Sodium: Sea Salt, Himalayan Pink Salt, Celery Salt, Vegetable Salt, Braggs Aminos Acids and Tamari. No soy sauce or iodized table salts.

Juices: Freshly squeezed – no sugar added, iced tea and hot teas – especially Green Tea.

Other: Organic Greek Yogurt, Feta cheese, and goat cheeses.

Eat foods that are whole, organic, not processed – REAL food. If you are going to do butter, eat real butter. If you are going to eat sugar, eat raw sugar or brown sugar. If you are going to eat meat, make sure it is not filled with hormones and antibiotics.

Oh! I almost forgot another lost superfood…Sourdough. Years ago a friend and excellent baker gave Jack a start of her 125 year old sourdough! He has been making pancakes ever since.☺ If you can get your hands on a start, do so.

Sourdough Benefits:
1. Glycemic Index Diet – Do you need to eat food low on the glycemic chart? Sourdough is a complex carbohydrate that converts to energy not fat. Sourdough breads are around 68 on the glycemic index compared to most other breads that are at 100.

2. Lactobacillus – Do you need some live enzymes in your gut to help aid digestion? Sourdough is brimming with lactobacillus, which is the most important of the bacteria found in sourdough. It produces lactic, formic and acetic acids which help prevent harmful organisms, including E. coli, from taking root.

3. Biotin – Do you need some vitamins? B-complex vitamins, such as biotin, are contained in sourdough. Biotin is an important element in cell growth, the metabolizing of fats and amino acids and the production of fatty acids.

To help you transition we included some of our favorite recipes in Chapter 12 are simple and tasty. I, Dani, include some time saving crockpot recipes; they are cooked but still provide nutritious meals on the run. A few recipes are from our family restaurant but do not tell my Mom...she holds them in a vault under lock and key.☺

So you change your diet, you exercise, you pick up a hobby, you spend time with friends and you do things that add to your life but it's still not enough. This was our experience for years. The reality is that America is the most overfed, malnourished country on the planet. We are also the most overmedicated. We live in a world that eats more "food stuffs" than we do REAL food. Raw fruits and vegetables are the highest in antioxidants, but according to a study done by UNICEF in 1992 (the most recent study I could find), our soils are more than 75% deficient in vitamins and minerals.[11] Even organic food may no longer supply our cells with the amount of basic building blocks and nutrients they need to maintain health so what is the solution?

In my opinion, and many others, the only solution to these dilemmas is to supplement our diet with plant-derived whole food supplements that contain a broad spectrum of antioxidants; fruits, vegetables, plants and herbs from every color of the rainbow. Supplementing is the fastest and easiest way to add these vital nutrients.

We have all heard the saying, "You are what you eat," but the reality is "We are what we absorb!" Healing is a process. First your body must arrest (stop) the progression of damage, then it can start repairing and regenerating health. Consistency is connected to healing. We must give our body these nutrients every day so it can naturally create health. Once our cells finally get the proper nutrients they can heal themselves but if the foods and the supplements do not have these vital nutrients, then how is your body going to get them?

We have learned a lot about supplements along the way. Even though people do experience total health transformations supplementing is for prevention and maintenance, not to treat or cure disease. Trial and error along with study has proven that not all supplements are 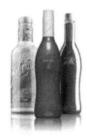 created equal as some contain mostly fillers or impure plant products and toxic ingredients. Sometimes, the plants from which the supplements are made were grown in soils that lack the necessary vitamins and minerals to create a plant rich in nutrition and photonic energy. In my opinion, many of the supplements, Chinese herbs, etc., that Jack had tried in the past just were not saturated or bioavailable enough for his cells to absorb and repair the damage done by sarcoidosis until Fucoydon and Spectramaxx. These were the two that really made a lasting difference for him.

As we shared earlier, Jack, and many other people with Sarcoidosis, have had excellent results adding a ½ to 1 ounce of Fucoydon, Spectramaxx and Eternity to their daily routine. Jack, me and our boys still take 1/2oz of Fucoydon every morning. Most of the time we just add it to a green smoothie!

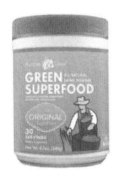

There are numerous wonderful green superfood powders that are organic, high in antioxidants, protein, and phytonutrients. Our favorite is organic Green Superfoods by Amazing Grass. Green SuperFood mixes well with juice or water but we add it to our Green smoothies. It includes a full spectrum of alkalizing green superfoods, antioxidant rich fruits, and support herbs with Acai and Maca to provide a powerful dose of whole food nutrition along with several natural TNF-a suppressors and a pro/prebiotic formula!

Green Superfoods:
• Helps you achieve your recommended daily servings of fruits and vegetables
• Naturally detoxifies and boosts your immune system
• Probiotics and Enzymes to aid digestion and absorption
• Complete raw food with powerful antioxidants
• Alkaline green plant foods balance acidic pH levels
• Contains over 70% organic ingredients, including tart cherry, green tea & broccoli
• More organic whole leaf greens per gram than other green superfoods - not from juice
• No soy lecithin fillers
• Nitrogen packed for freshness – this is very important. I will explain later.

Simply do a Google search for "green superfoods" and it will come up or you can find a link to order in the Resource Links in Chapter 12. Green Superfoods also contains tons of chlorella (excellent for alkalizing and detoxing the body) and some omegas, too! Their raw reserve is 100% organic, gluten free and vegan. It costs a bit more but you can buy it in bulk to get great discounts.

The active antioxidants, fucoidan, fulvic acid, quercetin, green tea, resveratrol and turmeric found in Fucoydon, Spectramaxx, Green Superfoods and Eternity are very beneficial nutrients for people with inflammatory autoimmune diseases and ones you should to consider adding to your daily regimen. We have researched many supplements containing these ingredients and tried to find the least costly, most effective options. The Green Superfoods powder is our favorite broad spectrum antioxidant option which contains green tea as well. We have yet to find any fucoidan supplement that compares to Fucoydon's concentration or cost. In total there are over 100,000 published studies on the nutrients in all four of these superfood supplements. Before Jack started taking Fucoydon and Spectramaxx I had never heard of fucoidan or fulvic acid but after Jack's results I was more than curious to find out about them both. I contribute 80% of Jack's amazing recovery to these two nutrients.

Fulvic Acid...A nutrient that heals!

Fulvic acid is referred to as "Nature's life force energy." This picture is the life force energy of a 'live' apple cut in half. Powerful stuff! So why do we not all know about it? Right?

Fulvic acid is a derivative of humeric substances that are a part of a decaying plant and animal matter. Extracted from the humeric substance, fulvic acid is the brown constituent of soil and is rich in nutrients and minerals. All food and nutrients supply chemical energy that is converted into electrical energy and fulvic acid or fulvates are the key that unlocks your body's ability to absorb all vitamins and minerals from foods and supplements.

Fulvic acid is invisible to the naked eye. They are microscopic electrolytes that empower all living organisms.[19] Their immense source of electrical energy supports revitalizing cell metabolism, a significant increase in organ respiration rates, and boosts overall health potential.[20]

Uses of fulvic acid include its antioxidant properties to remove free radicals from the body, as a buffer to help create an electrolyte balance within the body and to remove toxins from the body through its cleansing abilities.[21] Fulvic acid has also been used as a topical dressing for wounds, an antiviral treatment for shingles, athlete's foot and ringworm, and to neutralize the poisons in poison ivy and poison oak, which I just experienced for the first time after a five-day rafting trip. ☺

Fulvates are water-based organic electrolytes (substances that dissolves in water and are capable of conducting an electrical charge) composed of low-weight or small molecular substances secreted by microorganisms in the soil enabling plants to provide life force energy to plants and animals that eat them. So that is how we get the nutrients from the food we eat! We really are what we absorb.

Have you ever heard that your body will not use certain vitamins without the right amount of minerals, etc.? For minerals to be effectively utilized by living organisms, they must first be converted from their colloidal or metallic state to a microscopic subcolloidal or ionized state. Before being complexed or chelated with organic fulvic acid, large colloidal minerals and nutrients are in suspension-too large for easy absorption by living cells. Once complexed with organic fulvates, colloidal minerals and nutrients are dissolved in solution and are therefore more bioavailable. Maybe that's why they find all those whole vitamins in the sewers of America?!? The vitamins and minerals are too large for our cell to actually absorb.

Fulvates deliver vital nutrients to the gastrointestinal system, bloodstream & cells. They eliminate toxins from body & deliver substantial electrical energy, minerals and other nutrients to the body. As an acceptor, fulvates clear out toxins, energy depleted nutrients and exhausted minerals from the cell.[22] They also help build healthy & strong bone, enhance intestinal permeability to the minerals calcium, magnesium, iron, manganese, zinc and sulfate. Enhance skeletal health by supporting the natural body processes that utilize calcium and all minerals for strong bones.[23] (We often hear about calcium & Vit D with

Sarcoidosis. Studies show that 5-10% of people with Sarcoidosis have elevated vitamin D levels.[24] Before you take vitamin D supplements have a 1,25(OH)2D3 test to show if you have these complications.) In my opinion, the fulvic acid helped Jack properly assimilate all of these vitamins and minerals.

Fulvates promote smooth supple skin even when applied topically. Organic fulvic acid supports and maintains protein metabolism by mediating healing effects. It also helps support the body against the toxicity of known carcinogens.[25] You can simply purchase organic fulvic acid and add it to your daily regimen.

There are few known side effects associated with the use of fulvic acid. Starting therapy with a high dose may lead to some complaints of diarrhea for the first couple of days, but this usually subsides without any further problems. There have been no reports of dangerous side effects with the use of fulvic acid in either animals or humans.

For those considering taking Spectramaxx I will include the "must know" info. Spectramaxx is a broad spectrum supplement with 40 antioxidants, 74 essential trace minerals and Organic Fulvic Acid. Spectramaxx is formulated to neutralize free radicals and toxins. Science shows that the higher the Oxygen Radical Absorbance Capacity (ORAC) the greater power an antioxidant has to neutralize free radicals.26

Spectramaxx contains 40 extracts from all natural sources of vegetables, fruits and herbs. The combination will attack both the reactive oxygen species (ROS) and the reactive nitrogen species (RNS). With the air being about 80% nitrogen, antioxidants must be able to combat and protect against both.

ORAC Comparison Chart:

1. SpectraMaxx   5377 uM 1 oz
2. Noni juice   500 uM 1 oz
3. Acai juice   1310 uM 1 oz
4. Gogi Berry juice   400 uM 1 oz
5. Mangosteen   550 uM 1 oz

Spectramaxx contains super-saturated actives from: Plum, Grape, Black Currant, Blueberry, Raspberry, Chocolate, Lycium (Wolfberry), Goji, Grape Seed extract, Raspberry Seed extract, Cranberry, Prune, Tart Cherry, Wild Bilberry extract, Strawberry, Lime, Kiwi, Mango, Pomegranate, Mangosteen, Broccoli, Tomato, Carrot, Spinach, Kale, Brussel Sprout, Onion, Green Tea, White Tea, Coffee (bean) extract, Bilberry, Acai, Grape (skin) extract, Turmeric (root) extract, Sea Buckthorn (fruit) Puree, and Lemon (fruit) powder.

So we've covered two wonderful antioxidant supplements and the amazing power of fulvic acid. Now let's talk about my most favorite nutrient on the planet, fucoidan! As I shared before, Jack and our entire family, including the kids, take ½oz. (15ml) of a product called Fucoydon every morning. Fucoydon is formulated around the nutrient fucoidan.

What Is Fucoidan? Fucoidan is now thought to have a role to play in the stem cell-induced repair of cardiovascular damage. Fucoidan also stimulates an increase in levels of interferon gamma, which generates increased immune activity during infections and cancer states.[27-28] Furthermore, it can inhibit hyperplasia (abnormal cell overgrowth) in rabbits and induce apoptosis (programmed cancer cell death) in human lymphoma cell lines. [29-30] Studies show that fucoidan plays a role in the control of acute and chronic inflammation via selectin blockade, enzyme inhibition and inhibiting the complement cascade.[31] WOW, now that's a lot of info that I don't expect anyone to understand but just in case...I included it.

Fucoidan also contains the antioxidants necessary to help prevent the negative effects sustained from free radical damage, surprise, surprise! Researchers in Madrid, Spain, showed that ingredients in brown seaweed exhibited great capacity as a natural antioxidant -- even greater than extracts from green and red sea plants.

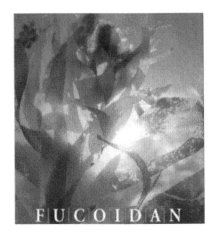

The Chinese have referred to fucoidan as "Virgin Mother's Milk" for centuries because it contains all the same nutrients and healing abilities as breast milk. Scientists know fucoidan as a "sulfated polysaccharide". This simply refers to the fact that this functional nutritional molecule is a complex of many sugars (poly = many, saccharide = sugar) with an element of sulfur attached. Since 1996, a total of four Nobel Prizes in medicine have been awarded for work in glycobiology (the study of sugar chains or glycans). Unlike other nutrients, fucoidan provides all eight saccharides (biological sugars), which have recently been identified as being absolutely essential for cell-to-cell communication through glycoproteins and glycolipids.

The main effective ingredient in fucoidan is the fucose, one of the eight essential biological sugars. Typically, only glucose and galactose are in the foods we eat so we do not consume fucose. We must produce over 34 different enzymatic reactions to generate intermediate molecules to make fucose. If there is any problem in any step (due to toxins, stress, etc.) during the conversion process, it will cause a severe and chronic disease.

Fucoidan contains all eight essential Saccharide's for cellular communication: Mannose, Glucose, Fucose, Galactose, N-acetylgalactosamine, N-acetylglucosamine, Xylose, and N-acetylneurominic acid. Below is a list of health benefits associated with each:

Mannose
- Prevents bacterial, viral, parasitic and fungal infections
- Eases inflammation in rheumatoid arthritis
- Lupus patients are deficient in this saccharide
- Lowers blood sugar and triglyceride levels in diabetic patients

Glucose

- Potent fast-energy source
- Enhances memory
- Stimulates calcium absorption
- Elderly Alzheimer's patients register lower levels of this saccharide than those with organic brain disease from stroke or other vascular diseases
- Glucose metabolism disturbed in depression, manic-depression, anorexia and bulimia

Fucose

- Increases growth factors IGF-1 and 2 identical to those found abundant in breast milk
- Influences brain development and ability to create long-term memories
- Induces production of immune factors interferon and interleukin in immunocytes
- Regulates immunomodulating activity
- Activates stem cells
- Creates hormonal anti-aging longevity factors
- Inhibits tumor growth through apopitosis
- Metabolism of this saccharide is abnormal in cystic fibrosis, diabetes, cancer and shingles
- Active against other herpes viruses, including herpes I and cytomegalovirus
- Guards against respiratory infections
- Inhibits allergic reactions by suppressing ige Increases growth factors for muscle rebuilding
- Stimulates bone growth and repair

- Creates growth factors for skin, hair, lining of internal organs
- Acts directly with anti-inflammatory inhibitors
- Re-pigments graying hair
- Potent energy metabolism increase
- Natural high ORAC value protects eyes and major organs

Galactose
- Enhances wound healing
- Increases calcium absorption
- Triggers long-term memory formation

N-Acetylgalactosamine
- Heart disease patients have lower-than- normal levels of this saccharide
- Inhibits spread of tumor
- Immune modulator with antitumor properties and activity against HIV

N-Acetylglucosamine
- Vital to learning
- Glucosamine, a metabolic product of this saccharide
- Helps repair cartilage
- Decreases pain and inflammation
- Increases range of motion
- Repair mucosal-lining defensive barrier implicated in Crohn's disease, ulcerative colitis and interstitial cystitis

N-Acetylneurominic Acid
- Important for brain development and learning
- Repels bacteria, virus and other pathogens
- Abundant in breast milk

Xylose
- Antibacterial and antifungal
- May prevent cancer of the digestive tract

Fucoidan side effects: Because of its anticoagulant property, fucoidan may have additive effects with anticoagulants such as warfarin and heparin. If you are on a prescription blood thinning medication you should consult your physician before taking fucoidan.

Adverse Reactions: No adverse reactions have been reported from the use of Fucoidan.[32]

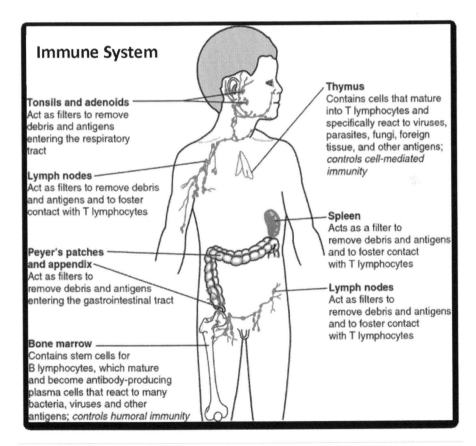

Before we learn more about how fucoidan activates intestinal immunity let's first learn about the importance of intestinal immunity. Intestinal immunity is referred to as the home of the Immune system. Our immune system attacks and defends against harmful external substances through the synergistic actions of various immune cells and bioactive substances such as Natural Killer (NK) cells, macrophages and interferons. Our bone marrow, thymic gland, spleen, lymph nodes and blood vessels are representative organs that contribute to the immune system. But the intestinal tract is the largest key of all. It is the largest organ in our body that provides immunity, called intestinal immunity. Our intestinal tract is the last defense against intrusion of foreign substances like toxins, pathogens, viruses, fungus, molds, and bacteria from getting introduced into our body.

Around 60% of all lymphocytes are in our intestinal tract. The surface of the small intestine is covered in 30 million or so "villi" (small finger-like projections that protrude from the epithelial lining of the intestinal wall). The surface of these villi consist of epithelial cells and T cells are between them. It is believed that these T cells monitor epithelial cells that frequently metabolize and detect if they have become cancerous. We all have cancer cells that form every day. To kill these cells, our intestinal tract (immunity) must be healthy. Once cancer cells are found, T cells will eliminate and destroy them much the same as they do with any mutated cell.

Capillaries run immediately below epithelial cells and the proper mucous membrane is found around these capillaries. T cells, B cells, and other lymphocytes are found in this membrane, creating an immune system in its own right. B cells exist in the greatest number among all lymphocytes in the membrane and function to synthesize Immunoglobulin A (IgA) antibody, a substance that works as a weapon against foreign substances by neutralizing harmful bacteria, viruses, and suppresses abnormal growth of inner-intestinal bacteria (bad bacteria, like candida, etc.). In the small intestine there is an immune tissue called a "Peyer's patch." The patch is the control tower of intestinal immunity controlling immune functions of the intestinal tract. Epithelial cells covering the patch are M cells. Everything that enters the small intestines is carried to the Peyer's patch by M cells. The patch macrophages check each substance to determine if it can be taken to the large intestine. If a foreign agent is found, helper T cells release cytokine and inform lymphocytes like natural killer cells, T cells and B cells, to attack the substance. Lymphocytes also form a barricade to keep pathogens from getting any further, into the blood stream, etc.

Since Sarcoidosis is an inflammatory, autoimmune-related disease, affecting the immune system, I thought you would appreciate this information. ☺

Finally – Fucoidan Mechanism of Action: Fucoidan is first introduced to the Macrophages or M cells that bring it to the Peyer's patch. Because fucoidan is a polysaccharide made of monosaccharide bonds that are not broken down in the stomach Macrophages mistake fucoidan for a harmful substance. When this complete polysaccharide gets to the small intestine, virtually intact, the Peyer's patch responds to it as a harmful substance. All lymphocytes attack it, which is a good thing because this activates lymphocytes and enhances our body's defense against pathogens.

Fucoidan diminishes the immune response and enhances the activity of NK cells, which play a crucial role in causing tumor cell death [33]. The neuroprotective effects of fucoidan are attributed to its ability to suppress tumor necrosis factor-alpha (TNF-a) and interferon-gamma (IFN-g) induced Nitric Oxide production in C6 glioma cells [34] and to its antioxidative effects.[35] Both of which are key to the progression and or suppression of inflammatory and autoimmune diseases.

Derived from ocean vegetation, fucoidan absorbs and holds water like a sponge; this property is responsible for the gooiness that is seaweed's most obvious characteristic. When sugar molecules are strung together in long polysaccharide chains it greatly enhances your body's ability to absorb water. This water trapping effect gives polysaccharides a slimy mucous quality that plays an important role in healing wounded biological tissues especially in the digestive system; basically coating and soothing inflamed and irritated digestive tissue not only calming and healing irritation, but just as importantly "sliming' away toxic substances like H-Pylori and other pesky bacteria as well as potentially problematic food particles (i.e. gluten and other allergy causing proteins).

The sulfur attachment to the polysaccharide provides benefits too. Formation of collagen, detoxification and activation of important biomolecules like cholesterol and Vitamin D are examples of sulfur dependent biological functions that can be enhanced by the cleavage of sulfur from its polysaccharide attachment in fucoidan. Finally, sulfur allows fucoidan to attach itself to various enzymes and tissues enhancing its biological activity even further. Obviously, we LOVE fucoidan and agree with leading researchers from around the world that state they have never seen one nutrient do more for the human body than fucoidan.

Four Things to Consider When Searching for a Fucoidan Supplement:

1. **Source:** In today's toxic and radiated environment you want to be sure the source/processing are radiation free. Contact the manufacturer to find out.
2. **Processing:** How is the fucoidan extracted? Is it bio-available and sulphated?
3. **Concentration:** For any nutrient to be effective it must be concentrated in a therapeutic dose.
4. **Cost:** I wish we never had to consider the cost when it comes to our health but let's face it – it can get expensive. When we were looking for a fucoidan supplement to help relieve inflammation due to

sarcoidosis, we called one company which formulated capsule and liquid. The seaweed was sourced from Japan which raised concern due to current events. The capsules were $300.00 a month and the liquid was $800.00 for one person. YIKES!

There are many fucoidan supplements available on the market. Just be sure to do your research. We chose a liquid supplement called Fucoydon which contains fucoidan sources from Tonga. There are 20 patent pending processes, some of which enzymatically cut the repeating fucoidan polysaccharide into smaller, individual molecules, maintaining the effective F, U and G individual molecules and adding sulfate groups to each molecule. This enhances absorption and concentrates the fucoidan without containing toxicity.

I just got this email the other day:

> "Yes, I am juicing (mostly vegetables - broccoli, asparagus, spinach, celery, and carrots) and I do find they make such a difference, too. I love it! ...and I have become all organized - separate them into bags prepped and ready to go so I only have to take the one bag out in the morning! I used to hate having to take them all out and going through them!
> Thanks to you, I am doing great! I did have to take Pulmicort last January when I got sick. I wore myself out during the holidays and got caught in a major snowstorm ...sheesh! I had a bad case of bronchitis, but apart from that, I feel terrific! And on

occasion, when I feel a little worn out, I take extra FuCoyDon, to make sure.

But really, I feel normal, at least, physically. Mentally...that is a whole other story. There has been a lot to deal with in the last three years, but now I am able to focus on things that make me happy.

I also love to seriously bike. I find it's great for my lungs. I will do about 45km in about two hours and I am working my way towards 50km plus in the same amount of time, although the weather has not been helpful.

Please believe me when I say that I am profoundly grateful. I realize I have said it before, but I do not think it can ever be said too often. I like to think that coming across your info on the web was divine intervention! Yep...Faith and FuCoyDon. They keep me smiling!

Well now, I have done it again - ANOTHER long email. lol!...and a BIG Italian hug to you!!!...which I will offer in person as I do hope to come to visit your restaurant in the not too distant future. You did say you have one, if I remember correctly.

Until then, all the very best! And kudos for the wonderful work you do!" Rosa

For over a year now Rosa has been faithfully altering her lifestyle to include juicing, regular exercise, fucoidan and things that bring her joy. She is creating harmony physically, mentally and spiritually. I love getting these emails – they make my week!

Another powerful nutrient worthy of mentioning is Resveratrol. If you are going to use a resveratrol supplement it is imperative that you know the information below before you waste your money.

Trans-Resveratrol vs. Cis-Resveratrol: In scientific studies, liquid Trans Resveratrol has been shown to trigger the sirtuins gene which controls functions in cells that lead to significant improvement in health which include: Anti-inflammatory, circulation and cardiovascular health, joint diseases, cancer, liver, macular degeneration, athletic endurance, acne, neurodegenerative diseases, Parkinson's, multiple sclerosis, Alzheimer's disease and more.[36] Resveratrol protects a cell's DNA and is a powerful antioxidant. [37]

Both trans-resveratrol and CIS-resveratrol are found naturally in Japanese Knotweed and red wine grapes. However, Trans-Resveratrol is the beneficial health substance in resveratrol products, while CIS has no health benefits. High purity resveratrol contains high amounts of trans-resveratrol, while lower purity products contain higher amount of CIS-resveratrol because it is the least expensive form.

When medicinal amounts of resveratrol are consumed, science has proven resveratrol significantly reduced oxidative stress levels in the brain and inhibits TNF-a, as stated earlier. Science has also shown that after seven days of consuming trans resveratrol, regeneration activity in the brain increased by 100% and regeneration of muscles, tissues and organs increased by 200%.[38] Resveratrol also creates more Mitochondria (the energy factories of the cells). In a study on resveratrol, scientists reported an increase in the number of mitochondria and enhanced motor activity levels.

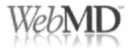

Red Wine Ingredient May Delay Aging

• Resveratrol May Prolong Life and Fight Age-Related Diseases

• Resveratrol is one of a group of antioxidant compounds called polyphenols found in red wine that has been reported to have anti-inflammatory as well as anticancer properties.

• Resveratrol, may counter type 2 diabetes and insulin resistance, a new study shows.

CNN -At high doses, resveratrol appears to prolong life spans and improve health in mice. Human trials are under way.

This research, funded in part by the National Institute on Aging, was published in the journals Nature and Cell in November, and bottles of resveratrol have been flying off the shelves since. Dr. Brent Bauer, director of the Department of Internal Medicine's Complementary and Integrative Medicine Program at Mayo Clinic says "This may be the best thing since sliced bread for human beings, but we just don't know yet."

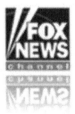

For years, red wine has been linked to numerous health benefits. But the new study, published online in the journal Nature on Thursday, shows that mammals given ultrahigh doses of resveratrol can get the good effects of cutting calories without actually doing it.

"If we're right about this, it would mean you could have the benefit of restricting calories without having to feel hungry," Sinclair said. "It's the Holy Grail of aging research."

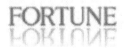

Resveratrol is the ingredient in red wine that made headlines in November when scientists demonstrated that it kept overfed mice from gaining weight, turned them into the equivalent of Olympic marathoners, and seemed to slow down their aging process. Few medical discoveries have generated so much instant buzz.

Drug interaction studies with resveratrol have not been conducted. People taking blood thinning medications such as aspirin, warfarin, or clopidogrel should advise their Dr. Additionally, you should always inform your health care providers of any dietary supplements or over-the-counter medications you use.

Patients who have blood disorders, which can cause bleeding, should be monitored by a physician while taking resveratrol. People undergoing surgery should stop taking resveratrol two weeks before the surgery and not take it for two weeks after the surgery to reduce the risk of bleeding. Do not take resveratrol supplements or excessive amounts of natural foods containing resveratrol while pregnant or breast-feeding. There is a lack of research in this area to prove safety. Resveratrol should be avoided in children.[39]

Resveratrol has mild estrogenic activity and until more is known, women with cancers and other conditions that are estrogen sensitive, should seek medical advice before taking resveratrol. Resveratrol reduces the activity of enzymes involved with drug metabolism, but whether it has a significant effect in humans has not been studied.[40]

Due to all the science thousands of resveratrol supplements have flooded the market in the last 3 years. Now you know the basics to consider when searching for an effective resveratrol supplement. Some of the ailments we've personally witnessed resveratrol help are psoriasis, Raynaud's, migraines, lupus, chronic fatigue, menopause and ALS.

Eterntity is one resveratrol product we are very familiar with and have used successfully in the past. Eterntiy is a liquid supplement containing resveratrol, quercetin and catechins. Should you choose to use Eternity here is some information to consider:

- Eternity uses 98–99% pure trans resveratrol from red grape seed and Japanese knotweed.
- One-half ounce serving of Eternity provides the resveratrol equivalent of 275 glasses of red wine.
- A blend of resveratrol plus quercetin, catechins, and other polyphenols work synergistically to maximize benefits.
- A proprietary liquid delivery system is designed to protect the Resveratrol blend through the entire digestive process and greatly enhance its cellular absorption.
- Eternity contains an energy blend made from Brazilian Cha-de-Bugre, grape skin, green tea, green coffee bean extracts, pomegranate, plum, and raspberry concentrates.

One IMPORTANT tip when taking any liquid resveratrol product is to hold it in your mouth for 60 seconds. This can increase absorbency by as much as 250%.

WOW, is your head spinning with all this information? We've only covered 4 great supplements with 100's of excellent ingredients that have helped 1000's of people with a multitude of different ailments, but there is an entire world of supplement options out there for you to choose from. It was important to us that we share exactly what

Jack and many others are using so you could make a more informed decision. You may have more questions and you can always email us, but please remember, these statements have not been evaluated by the FDA. These products are not intended to diagnose, treat, cure, or prevent any disease. We are not doctors and do not give medical advice. We simply share this information in hopes that it will offer additional options and help you make a more informed decision for your own health.

Chapter 8 Trivia: Why Do I Feel Worse Before I Feel Better?

I know you don't want to hear this but you may feel worse before you feel better. This is not always the case, but a wonderful friend of mine, Deirdre, whom I met because her entire family was diagnosed with Lyme disease more than 9 years ago, informed me of the Herxheimer Reaction, also referred to as the "die-off effect."

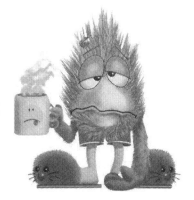

The Herxheimer Reaction is a short-term (from days to a few weeks) detoxification reaction in the body. As the body detoxifies, it is not uncommon to experience flu-like symptoms including headache, joint and muscle pain, body aches, sore throat, general malaise, sweating, chills, nausea or other symptoms.

When fighting an illness in the body, whether it be a cold, flu, infection, sarcoidosis or even cancer, protocols we implement such as herbs, broad spectrum antioxidants, fucoidan , cleansing, massage, acupuncture, sauna, essential oils, homeopathy, etc., may all result in a "die-off effect" of the culprit. This is also true for traditional or allopathic courses of healing such as chemotherapy, cold and sinus medicines, or prescribed antibiotics, corticosteroids and other medications. The resulting "die-off effect" of the pathogen is what you want. If the method used is capable of destroying a malignancy, a parasitic infiltration, or a systemic infection, the body has a need to carry off the toxic debris.   If we do not get rid of the toxins quickly enough for the body, lymph channels can become thick and blocked, sometimes resulting in metastases – the spread of a disease from one organ or part to another non-adjacent organ or part.

Herx "healing" Reaction	Drug or Other "allergy" Reaction
Delayed reaction	Immediate or quick reaction
Worsening of current symptoms	New symptom(s)
Accompanied by detoxification symptoms such as headache, muscle/joint aches & pains, sore throat, malaise, fever, nausea, hives or flu like symptoms	
Symptoms will calm down as the body slowly as the body gets on top of the detoxification process	Symptoms often resolve quite quickly
Symptoms are cyclic and usually flare in patterns of every 4 weeks (and often in conjunction with menses for females) with the worst of the herx often occurring at the fourth week of treatment.	Symptoms will be gone if the treatment or allergy producing item is removed or dose is decreased/changed in the case of medications e.g. antibiotics.

The Herxheimer's effect is your body's reaction to the overabundance of dead or dying bacteria, fungus, yeast, and viruses as a result of your treatment or protocol. The reaction carries with it a multitude of unpleasant side effects, including fatigue, diarrhea, headaches or migraines, muscle and joint aches, ringing in the ears, mental dullness and disorientation, and flu-like symptoms. This reaction is not counterproductive or a counter action of the process. It is your body telling you to flush the toxins more quickly.[41]

Russ McMillan, D.D.S., D.P.H., MD, P.H. suggests something that helps with the rather debilitating symptoms that accompany the Herxheimer effect after medication: Take a salts bath which consists of one cup salt, one cup soda, one cup Epsom salts, and one cup aloe vera, added to a hot bath. Remain in and keep hot for about 1 ½ hours, while consuming about two quarts of warm water. Evidently the perspiration and osmotic pressure removes the causative toxins.

This method, or the use of a dry or hot steam sauna, may help during cleansing or during the weaning time from prednisone. Fucoidan and fulvic acid can also be helpful, as they both chelate and pull toxins from the body, as well as, aid adrenal function.

Here is an excerpt from Deirdre's family results once they added fucoidan (you can read the entire story on her blog; www.LymeInChronicIllness.com.

"One day I was researching online, and listened in on Dani's radio show, and heard her tell the story about her husband Jack, and how he went into remission from sarcoidosis after several months using fucoidan. I have read that lyme can be the cause of sarcoidosis, and had suspected that my older son might even have it, due to his constant, unexplained shortness of breath and a couple of granulomas spotted on his lungs a few years ago on a chest CT scan. So we decided to give it a try. After nine months, taking a half-ounce to 1 ounce a day on an empty stomach, my husband and two older children and I retested our CD 57, and the levels for the first time ever improved significantly. And our symptoms began to greatly improve over that same period of time. Alexandra went from 18 CD 57 to 60. Keller went from 32 up to 84. My husband Jay went from 30 to 88! I tested mine after only three months on fucoydon and I went from 30 to CD 59."

Chapter 9: Anything But Conventional!

"The significant problems we have cannot be solved at the same level of thinking with which we created them." Albert Einstein

Isn't that the statement above so true?! We try and try to solve our issues using the exact same methods which got us here in the first place!

We have to change the way we think for anything else in our lives to change.   Due to the information age we live in and the vast ability to connect with people all over the world through social media, our world is wakening. We are part of empowering a paradigm.

It Is Time for Empowering a Paradigm!

Chronic Disease Statistics:

- In 2003, Dr. Allen Roses, international vice president of Glaxo-SmithKline one of the major drug manufactures in the world, admitted in a public interview, "The vast majority of drugs – more than 90% – only work on 30% to 50% of the people."
- Correctly prescribed medications make over 2 million people sicker every year, killing over 100,000 people yearly, while mistakes involving prescription medicines kills another 100,000 a year.
- About 133 million Americans, nearly 1 in 2 adults, live with at least one chronic illness.

- More than 75% of health care costs are due to chronic conditions.
- Approximately one-fourth of people living with a chronic illness experience significant limitations in daily activities.
- The percentage of U.S. children and adolescents with a chronic health condition has increased from 1.8% in the 1960s to more than 15% in 2011, and the percentage continues to climb.
- "Chemotherapy is only effective in 2% of cancers, in addition to reducing the remaining quality and length of life, and over 50% of those few who are supposedly "cured" by chemotherapy, develop secondary cancers from the chemotherapy and biopsies," stated Ralph Moss, Ph.D. & Life Extension Foundation's Scientific Advisory Board member
- "Chronic diseases—such as heart disease, cancer, and diabetes—are the leading causes of death and disability in the United States. Chronic diseases account for 70% of all deaths in the U.S., which is 1.7 million each year. Although chronic diseases are among the most common and costly health problems, they are also along the most preventable." Centers For Disease Control (Sarcoidosis is a chronic disease)

In a time when Americans are the most overfed, malnourished, medicated and unhealthy society in the world, we need to start empowering a paradigm. Health care (sickness care) costs exceeded $1.8 trillion last year and for some reason cancer, diabetes and heart disease are STILL on the rise.

So far, we have shared diet, supplementing, thermography, hydration, colonics, yet the world of wellness has so much more to offer. If main stream medicine will not speak of the power of nutrition, positive thinking, exercise, proper hydration, etc., to prevent chronic disease, we will happily scream it from the mountain tops.

According to *The Center For Managing Chronic Disease*, Chronic Disease is a long-lasting condition that can be controlled but not cured. But who says they're right? We used to think the Earth was round...what an ignorant and close minded thought!

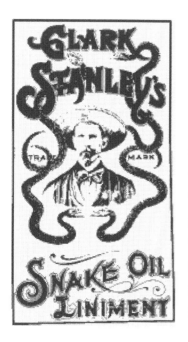

Whether you like change or not, let's be honest with ourselves, nobody wants status quo! We must get rid of all these limiting beliefs and do whatever it takes to NOT be a statistic. In this chapter we will cover hair analysis, toxic food syndrome, low level laser therapy, castor oil pack and skin soothing remedies but we hope that this book only wets your appetite, causing you to get curious and open your mind to more possibilities.

We probably should have started with hair analysis and toxic food testing, but these ideas came into our lives long after Jack had already started to recover. I will warn you that when you research any or ALL of these alternatives, you will certainly find contradicting information. Some swear by these methods and others call them 'quackery' but we've been sure to read the medical/scientific journals, articles and re-evaluate every single aspect of the information we have shared. We know how serious this subject is and how sick people are.

As I always say, question everything, consider the source and confirm the results. If you ask me, the powers that be are not going to expose the truth about these alternatives; for fear that it may just put them out of business.

Hair Tissue Mineral Analysis: Hair analysis came up briefly throughout my radio career, but we never covered it in detail. I wish we would have because my Mom recently used laser treatment (we will talk about that later) to help her Trigeminal Neuralgia and was told that heavy metal toxicity and corticosteroid use would interfere with the efficacy of treatment. They recommended she have hair tissue mineral analysis done.

Hair tissue mineral analysis, or HTMA, is a soft tissue mineral biopsy that uses hair as the sampling tissue. Hair is considered a soft tissue, and hence hair analysis is a soft tissue biopsy. The test measures the levels of 20 or more minerals and toxic heavy metals in the hair with an accuracy of plus or minus about 3%. This is about the same level of accuracy as most blood tests.[42]

A hair tissue mineral analysis can provide pertinent information about your metabolic rate, energy levels, sugar and carbohydrate tolerance, stage of stress, immune system and glandular activity and is a standard test used around the world for the biological monitoring of trace elements and toxic metals in humans and animals. The same technology is used for soil testing and testing of rock samples to detect mineral levels.[34]

Hair, like all other body tissues, contains minerals that are deposited as the hair grows.

Although the hair is dead, the minerals remain as the hair continues to grow out. A sample of hair cut close to the scalp provides information about the mineral activity in the hair that took place over the past three to four months, depending on the rate of hair growth.

My Mom's hair analysis report was 23 pages long and showed her mineral deficiencies, metabolic information and levels of several heavy metals. For anyone wondering what they are high or low in, this is the perfect test to start with and for under $200 you can get the test and a consultation with the physician.

Toxic Food Testing: (Listen to "Toxic Food Syndrome" with Immunolabs Founder Jeffrey Zavik): Have you ever had a doctor guarantee your results? Sounds too good to be true? Well, listen to the audio, "Toxic Food Syndrome," with Immuno Laboratories founder Jeffrey Zavik.

His life is another inspiring story about overcoming illness which drove his desire to start Immuno Laboratories and help millions of people around the world figure out which of the right foods were wrong for them.

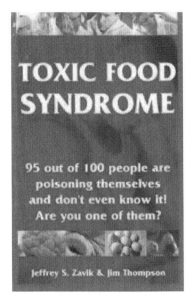

I encourage you to go to www.Immunolabs.com and check out the resource section where they share excellent recipes, articles and videos that can help you in your recovery. You can also go to www.sendmethefreebook.com and download his book, "Toxic Food Syndrome," for free. He was kind enough to offer it to our listeners when Dr. Powell and I had our show. According to Jeffrey, "95% of the people we have tested show that one or more foods they regularly eat cause a toxic reaction in their body."

You might not even notice these toxic reactions. Most of them work at a cellular level, and may cause symptoms that you will not notice right away. Or, you might not ever make the connection that what you are eating is actually damaging your body.

Nutritious foods that you eat like corn, egg whites, green pepper, cinnamon, whey, or chicken, for example, may actually act like a poison in your body. When you eat foods that form toxins in your system, those foods can cause harmful, chronic problems with your health. Remember earlier in the book we talked about our son Trent having serious stomach aches for almost a year while we took him back and forth to the doctor. Some of his other symptoms were leg aches, a chronic cough, runny nose, dark circles under his eyes, swollen lymph nodes and headaches. A food intolerance test revealed that it was all due to potato intolerance!

Immunolabs performs a specific bloodprint test. Years ago scientists discovered your body has an internal chemical balance that is as unique to you as your fingerprint. Likewise, every food you eat has its own "chemical balance" – a unique set of natural or man-made chemicals. As your body reacts differently to each and every food, the food you eat each day will enhance proper body chemistry, or disrupt the correct balance. One way to measure how your body reacts to the foods you eat is through the Bloodprint test, which pinpoints the foods that support healthy body chemistry and those that are toxic to you.

A food intolerance test is an absolute must for everyone and the first question I ask when people contact me is "Have you had a food intolerance test?"

Low Level Laser Therapy (LLLT): As I mentioned before, my Mom used LLLT to successfully relieve her TN pain. She went to a clinic in South Carolina called Curalase. To my knowledge there are many LLLT clinics around the country and many kinds of lasers. Some lasers are extremely powerful and others will not penetrate far enough to have any result so your homework.

In researching LLLT, I found this abstract on www.pubmed.gov: "Soon after the discovery of lasers in the 1960s, it was realized that laser therapy had the potential to improve wound healing, reduce pain, inflammation and swelling. In recent years, the field sometimes known as photobiomodulation has broadened to include light-emitting diodes and other light sources. The range of wavelengths used now includes many in the red and near infrared.

The term "low level laser therapy" or LLLT, has become widely recognized and implies the existence of the biphasic dose response called the Arndt-Schulz curve. This review will cover the mechanisms of action of LLLT at a cellular and at a tissular level, and will summarize the various light sources and principles of dosimetry that are employed in clinical practice. The range of diseases, injuries, and conditions that can be benefited by LLLT will be summarized with an emphasis on those that have reported randomized controlled clinical trials. Serious life-threatening diseases such as stroke, heart attack, spinal cord injury, and traumatic brain injury may soon be amenable to LLLT therapy."

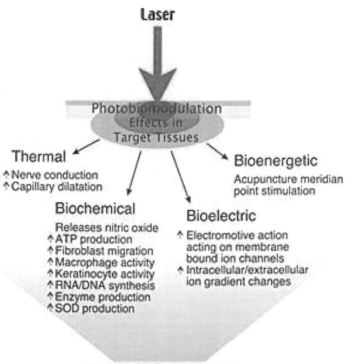

Laser

Photobiomodulation Effects in Target Tissues

Thermal
↑ Nerve conduction
↑ Capillary dilatation

Bioenergetic
Acupuncture meridian point stimulation

Biochemical
Releases nitric oxide
↑ ATP production
↑ Fibroblast migration
↑ Macrophage activity
↑ Keratinocyte activity
↑ RNA/DNA synthesis
↑ Enzyme production
↑ SOD production

Bioelectric
↑ Electromotive action acting on membrane bound ion channels
↑ Intracellular/extracellular ion gradient changes

CLINICAL EFFECTS

• Reduced spasm • Pain relief • Increased circulation
• Improved flexibility and function • Improved healing
• Reduced symptoms associated with osteoarthritis

The human body contains trillions of cells which are functional units for all living things. Each cell is an amazing world unto itself. It can take in nutrients, convert nutrients into energy, perform many special functions and reproduce itself. Each cell stores its own set of instructions and energy for carrying out specific activities.

Clinical evidence around the world demonstrates that laser energy stimulates the function of the cell in several ways. This evidence indicates: Laser energy is electromagnetic waves of energy carrying bundles of energy called photons.

The cells are capable of absorbing this energy directly into the Krebs cycle. This higher state of energy enhances the function of the cell. Other cellular responses include increased permeability and elasticity of the cell walls, allowing fluid that is trapped between the cells (lymphedema/inflammation) to flow back into the system and out through the natural waste processes. This often gives immediate improvement in range of motion and relief to joint pain and pitting edema. This improved elasticity also allows the blood vessels to dilate, thus increasing blood flow. The increased blood flow in the capillaries produces relief to the burning, stinging discomfort of neuropathic pain and facilitates faster wound healing.

Laser energy stimulates cells, including undifferentiated lymphocyte cells, to a higher level of activity. These unique cells can transform into many different kinds of cells, including phagocyte cells that miraculously appear at the site of an injury to clean the area. Undifferentiated lymphocyte cells can become bone, skin, muscle or most kinds of tissue needed. When the underlying condition is resolved, the pain is also resolved

LOW LEVEL LASER THERAPY (LLLT) OR NSAIDS (Nonsteroidal anti-inflammatory drugs):
NSAIDS are slow healing and often have side effects, whereas LLLT is non-invasive and improves healing, as well as, reducing inflammation and pain. Over 200 LLLT clinical trials (RCTs) and over 1,000 laboratory studies have been published. It has proven more effective and safer than pharmaceutical anti-inflammatories across a range of

musculoskeletal conditions. LLLT also improves healing and reduces muscle fatigue, muscle damage and Delayed Onset Muscle Soreness (DOMS).

"The use of low levels of visible or near infrared light for reducing pain, inflammation and edema, promoting healing of wounds, deeper tissues and nerves, and preventing cell death and tissue damage has been known for over forty years." Professor Michael Hamblin, Harvard-MIT Division of Health Sciences and Technology.

LLLT is also FDA approved for treating pain and most widely used by chiropractors and pain clinics. Considering my Mom's results and many others, I think this is a great therapy to consider especially for pain reduction. You can even purchase a laser for home use.

Castor Oil Packs - Relieve pain, inflammation and soften scar tissue: Don't worry you don't have to drink it! Thank goodness. In my experience, castor oil packs have helped with back pain, knee and ankle pain, Indigestion, irregularity and more. A castor oil pack is placed on the skin to increase circulation and to promote elimination and healing of the tissues and organs underneath the skin. They are used to stimulate the liver, relieve pain, increase lymphatic circulation, reduce inflammation, and improve digestion.

Castor oil packs are a traditional holistic treatment for a range of conditions, such as: cholecystitis (inflammation of the gall bladder), poor eliminations, epilepsy, various liver conditions such as cirrhosis and torpid liver, scleroderma, headaches, appendicitis, arthritis, colitis, intestinal disorders such as stricture and colon impaction, incoordination between nervous systems, neuritis, and toxemia.

To make a castor oil pack, you will need the following:
- High quality cold-pressed castor oil
- A hot water bottle or heating pad
- Plastic wrap, sheet of plastic, or plastic garbage bag
- Two or three one-foot square pieces of wool or cotton flannel, or one piece that is large enough to cover the entire treatment area when folded in thirds
- One large old bath towel

Castor Oil Pack Instructions: (courtesy of Daniel H. Chong, ND):
- Fold flannel three layers thick so it is still large enough to fit over your entire upper abdomen and liver, or stack the three squares.
- Soak flannel with the oil so that it is completely saturated. The oil should be at room temperature.
- Lie on your back with your feet elevated (using a pillow under your knees and feet works well), placing the flannel pack directly onto your abdomen; cover oiled flannel with the sheet of plastic, and place the hot water bottle on top of the plastic.
- Cover everything with the old towel to insulate the heat. Take caution not to get the oil on whatever you are laying on, as it can stain. If necessary, cover that surface with something to protect it.

- Leave pack on for 45 to 60 minutes.
- When finished, remove the oil from your skin by washing with a solution of two tablespoons of baking soda to one quart water, or just soap and water. (Be sure to wash the towel by itself, as the castor oil can make other clothes stink if washed together.)
- You can reuse the pack several times, each time adding more oil as needed to keep the pack saturated. Store the pack in a large zip-lock bag or other plastic container in a convenient location, such as next to your bed. Replace the pack after it begins to change color.
- For maximum effectiveness, apply at least four consecutive days per week for one month. Patients who use the pack daily report the most benefits.

As with everything else, you must be careful about your source of castor oil. Much of the oil currently sold in stores is derived from castor seeds that have been heavily sprayed with pesticides, solvent-extracted (hexane is commonly used), deodorized, or otherwise chemically processed, which damages beneficial phytonutrients and may even contaminate the oil with toxic agents.

Tip: If you can find it, Rosa Mosqueta oil is a little known secret to remove scar tissue, but buy it pure. Gently rub it in before applying the castor oil pack so the oleic and linoleic acids in the oil can start to replace scar tissue (collagen webbing) with normal cells, collagen and elastin.

There are so many alternative therapies we have not even talked about yet: meditation, yoga, acupuncture, essential oils, and homeopathy. We encourage you to do your own research. As we learn we will continue to share new discoveries as well. Be sure to refer to the resources section in chapter 12 for all the links, online ordering, books, etc., we have talked about. Know that healing is one step at a time.

Natural skin soothing and healing remedies: Below you will find many options for soothing skin rashes, sores, wounds, etc. Sarcoidosis often time affects the skin, causing rashes, irritation, itchiness, dryness, open wounds, and more. Below are before and after pictures along with an email from Keith, a friend and sarcoidosis survivor, who wanted to share his results using Tea Tree oil.

"In summer of 2012, my head developed an open wound. It had done this the previous year as well and stuck around for approximately three months and would not heal. I tried ointments and peroxide. No help. It then went away in late fall on its own. In January of this year, it started again. I then tried applying tea tree oil to the open sore and within three weeks it was gone.

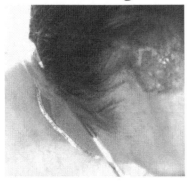 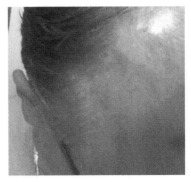

Wow, it worked. Amazing! I used a q-tip and applied it in the evening before bed and once again in the morning after a shower. Just wanted to share this with fellow sarcoidosis sufferers. Hope it works for everyone else, too."

Keith

Tea Tree oil: has become a popular natural ingredient in all kinds of shampoos, face soaps and ointments because of its amazing healing powers. Australian aboriginals have known the secret to healthy glowing skin for centuries. They used Tea Tree oil to soothe skin and to heal cuts, ring worm and athlete's foot, soften corns, cuts and scrapes, itching of insect bites and chicken pox, warts, acne, dandruff, and we can now add sarcoidosis to this list!

Tea Tree oil can also treat minor wounds, encourage healing, and prevent infection.
Below are additional emollients you may want to try. Emollients are the key ingredients in skin care that soothe and protect irritated or inflamed skin, moisturize, and help replenish the skin's natural oils. When used topically on the skin, herbs that are rich in mucilage are called emollients. Natural vegetable, nut and seed oils are emollients that lubricate and help skin remain smooth and pliable. Emollients are important to those with serious skin disorders such as, psoriasis and eczema, as well as, anyone with dry, irritated or aging skin.

Almond Oil: Used in skin care and aromatherapy as a carrier oil. Raw almonds are used in facial scrubs, and to make almond flour and almond butter.

Aloe Vera: The leaf juices of the aloe plant have important medicinal uses, making Aloe one of the most respected medicinal plants found in many gels, creams and lotions. We use Aloe Vera juice in our green smoothies. Yum!

Other benefits include:

- Halts the growth of cancer tumors.
- Lowers high cholesterol.
- Repairs "sludge blood" and reverses "sticky blood."
- Boosts the oxygenation of your blood.
- Eases inflammation and soothes arthritis pain.
- Protects the body from oxidative stress.
- Prevents kidney stones & protects the body from oxalates in coffee and tea.
- Alkalizes the body, helping to balance overly acidic dietary habits.
- Helps ulcers, IBS, Crohn's disease and other digestive disorders.
- Reduces high blood pressure naturally by treating the cause, not just the symptoms.
- Nourishes the body with minerals, vitamins, enzymes and glyconutrients.
- Accelerates healing from physical burns and radiation burns.
- Makes bandages and antibacterial sprays obsolete.
- Halts colon cancer, heals the intestines and lubricates the digestive tract.
- Stabilizes blood sugar and reduces triglycerides in diabetics.
- Prevents and treats candida infections.

- Protects kidneys from disease.
- Functions as nature's own "sports drink" for electrolyte balance.
- Boosts cardiovascular performance and physical endurance.
- Speeds recovery from injury or physical exertion.
- Hydrates the skin and accelerates skin repair.

After reading the health benefits of this one plant, I hope you go get an Aloe plant. You can use the Aloe from the leaves topically and fillet it to get the gel out and use in smoothies, juices, drinks and in other recipes as well.

Castor Oil: Apply castor oil externally for muscle and arthritis pain, bruising and nerve damage. It is well suited to the slow relief of chronic pain and swelling.

Coconut Oil: Works wonders for dry and damaged skin, cuts, bruises, and speeds healing while it fights infection.

Comfrey salves, ointments and teas: Best known for the topical treatment of burns and just about any skin irritation.

Slippery Elm: In herbal medicine, slippery elm bark powder is considered one of the best poultices for wounds, boils, ulcers, burns and reducing pain and inflammation.
Jojoba Oil: Absorbs into the skin so well that there is no greasy or tacky feel to it. Known for its ability to smooth fine lines and wrinkles, Jojoba Oil rejuvenates and rehydrates dry skin.

Neem Oil: Rich, thick and protective of skin and hair. Use it as a topical treatment for athlete's foot, scabies and any fungal infections of the skin.

Oatmeal Extract: The liquid left from cooking whole oats is one of the most soothing and effective treatments for dry skin and sunburns, and can help heal damage from more serious skin conditions, such as serious eczema and psoriasis.

Sea Buckthorn Oil: Used in healing skin injuries, burns, wounds, eczema, lesions, sun damaged skin, and abrasions.

Shea Butter: Rich in vitamins, minerals and fatty acids that rejuvenate and hydrate skin and hair. Use Shea Butter to treat damaged skin, help heal wounds, or just pamper yourself.

Chapter 10: Mind Over Matter – Outwitting Sarcoidosis
written by Jack Walker

"90% of the game is half mental." John Madden

I, Jack, would not allow myself to be confined by traditional methods and have always been an 'out-of-the box' kind of thinker. That also applies to my thought process when battling Sarcoidosis. I agree with Dani; it is time to empower a paradigm!

The saying, "up a creek without a paddle," actually means you are in an unfortunate situation, unprepared and with none of the resources to remedy the matter. What is it like to be alone in the wilderness without even a compass, having to find your way by the moss growing on the north side of the trees? When it comes to Sarcoidosis, I sure felt like I was lost, alone, unprepared with no resources to remedy the matter. The doctors were all looking for answers just like I was. When your sherpa loses their way it is easy to lose hope yourself. I often felt that I knew more about my disease than my doctors did. They never once suggested any dietary changes, exercise, rest, meditation. Anything that was outside of surgery and medication was up to me to figure out.

My mental attitude started with small incremental steps of positivity on a daily basis, especially in the beginning when I did not "feel" like it. There were times when having sarcoidosis in my lymph, heart and lungs was more than overwhelming but to realized that harnessing the power of my mind was the beginning of crawling out of this dark place. I had to take my thoughts captive and let go of any limiting beliefs.

Even when I was in pain and could not move, I had to find something good about my life and build on it. After trying Western medicine for three years, I had to think 'outside the prescription' as my wife Dani would say. This is where I believe that having the mindset of the victor instead of the victim helped me most. I looked at it as any other fight in my life. I would not be defeated. I believe that we are all divine and should not just acept the opinions of even highly educated people if it does not resonate in our soul.

Everyone has an opinion and they will give it to you whether you want it or not, but nobody, and I do mean nobody, knows what the future holds for you or me. We truly do create our own realities: we can either overcome the problem or become the problem. I never said that I had sarcoidosis and always looked at it as something that was leaving my body. This was the thought process that kept my mind open to other alternatives that eventually led to my remission.

For instance, when doctors told me I would not lose the weight I had gained from prolonged prednisone use that damaged my thyroid, I continued to cycle anyway. I set out to do what could not be done. Just like with positive thoughts, I started small, riding five to six miles and after remission, working my way up to 70 mile rides. I currently ride 20-40 miles two or three times a week.

I have always been the type of person that if you tell me it cannot be done, I will do it just to prove you wrong. So if you are not that type of person feel free to borrow this attitude from me! I feel it is the biggest factor to overcoming anything in life, especially sickness and Sarcoidosis.

There have been so many great things that have come from this disease. I used to be so driven for success that I would work 70 hours a week, all the while missing my children growing up. When I was home, I would fertilize, water and mow until our lawn looked like Fenway Park. You know -- trying to keep up with the Jones. The beauty of a life threatening illness is that, at least for me, it gave me perspective on what is really important in life. Who cares if the kids leave a few toys in the yard and the clean dishes are not put away.

It was no longer exciting to have a 180 MPH sport bike. It was time to prioritize and spend time with my loved ones; the people sticking by me through this battle. Spending time camping, floating on the rivers, going to baseball games, never missing one of the boys' sporting events, learning to appreciate all the beauty around me and literally stopping to smell the roses became far more important than shear speed!

At the same time, I had the honor of seeing my wife flourish with her new found passion to help people overcome seemingly incurable diseases. As you know, she started a blog, helping people all over the world which led to a radio show and many amazing friendships. I've watched her shed many tears, share much joy an encourage so many survivors over the years.

We have met so many courageous people that share similar values and refuse to settle for anything less than victory. Even if it is just a listening and understanding ear, it is such an honor to be able to encourage people. We understand that many people do not make themselves available but for Dani and me it always seems strange how shocked people are when we answer the phone or respond to emails. Why wouldn't we? To help people overcome seemingly incurable disease is our mission.

Believe in yourself and your body's ability to heal and learn to trust your intuition. If it is not right for you, it will not "feel" right for you. You were placed on this earth to be a victor, not a victim, so take your personal power back from anyone who tells you different. Together we all make a difference.

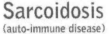

Sarcoidosis
(auto-immune disease)

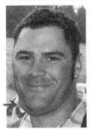

Before

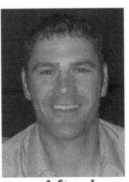

After!

"Collectively our courage can change the face of Sarcoidosis."
Jack Walker

Chapter 10 Trivia by Dani Walker: What is your "Freak"Quency? (Listen to "What Is EFT?" audio)

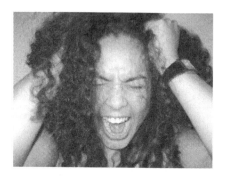

After Jack wrote this chapter I felt it very fitting to talk about the power of the mind, emotions, thoughts, etc.

We are spiritual beings having a human experience. Life is to have experience of the "emotion." An excellent documentary about this is called *What the Bleep Do We Know?* Emotions have a frequency and what is eating you is just as important as what you are eating. Each emotion has a vibration: shame and guilt are very low, freezing us into "no action." Love is very high, and gratitude and compassion are the highest vibrations.

Your brain is a pharmacy that is open 24/7 made up of 78% water and 60% good fat. As I stated before, at the chemical level, food is the brain's primary link to its environment and to its evolution. Your diet affects the brain chemicals that influence your mood and behavior: the thought processes and emotional reactions that ultimately create the story of our lives.

The human body has 28 different kinds of amino acids and brain tissue is made up of neuro-transmitters which need amino acids and nutrients to function efficiently. Neuro-peptides are called the 'Molecules of Emotions' and seventy percent of the neuro-peptides in the human body line the inside and outside of the gastro-intestinal track. There are

100 different kinds of neuro-peptides and they all exist in the brain AND the heart! They are individually all over the body squirting an enzyme of hormone depending on what they "feel" from the vibrations of incoming food and emotions. These neuro-peptides do not need a direct signal from the brain. Your heart-felt emotions are real; your gut instincts are true!

We have the ability to change our environment, our thoughs, fears, etc. and one of the most interesting techniques I've ever learned is Emotional Freedom Technique. Emotional Freedom Technique (EFFT) is also referred to as "Tapping" and is a method of helping you overcome negative emotions, pain, etc. EFT is so effective that the medical community is embracing it as a treatment for Post-Traumatic-Stress-Syndrome.

Emotional Freedom Technique: (Listen to audio "What is EFT?")

As you listen to the audio I would like to set the stage for you. My radio show was totally mine, to plan, to market, to find guests, to promote, to take care of and on this very day I had a different guest speaker scheduled. I had planned the entire one hour show around a specific healing modality, with a special 'Guru' guest. I was 'sitting pretty' when 20 minutes before the show aired LIVE, my cell rang.

You guessed it; they canceled on me last minute! How rude and irresponsible to just leave me hanging like that. But, life happens so we adapt and overcome, RIGHT!!!!! I started making calls to my circle of 'outside the prescription thinkers' and my dear friend Marla came to the rescue. Actually, because she came to the rescue she became my dear friend. Before this show I had briefly talked to her on the phone once. I had no idea what Emotional Freedom Technique was, Marla and I were totally 'free style' and the show was a blast! Listen and enjoy the information.

EFT Tapping stands for "The Emotional Freedom Techniques." EFT Tapping is also referred to as "emotional acupuncture" or *acupuncture for the emotions without the needles*. The more modern Emotional Freedom Techniques use some of the same areas for Tapping as the ancient Chinese acupuncture utilizes. The areas or points, are a part of the energetic field in the body known as the meridian system.

Medical science has finally grasped the significance of mindset and emotional wellness in healing the physical body. More and more research points to the fact that Energy Medicine is strongly effective in changing the brain's chemistry, therefore improving the body's ability to heal.

EFT Tapping is based on the theory that the cause of all negative emotions is a disruption in the body's energy system. As we go through life we take on beliefs and understandings as a result of our experiences and exposure to the thoughts and actions of others. Some of those beliefs and thought patterns may be strongly negative, causing varying levels of trauma to our energy system and eventually cause a blockage in the flow of energy through the meridian system. Much like how our arteries carry blood through our body, the meridian system carries our energy. When there are blockages of this energy the result is negative emotion, distress, and eventually physical illness may even occur.

How Does EFT work?
The Discovery Statement in EFT is: *"The cause of all negative emotions is a disruption in the body's energy system."* It is theorized that by tapping the acupuncture meridians these disruptions can be reduced or eliminated. That is what causes the positive shifts in emotions. What is the first thing you do when you are confronted with painful, threatening or negative circumstances? Typically we freeze: our minds race, our pulse quickens, and our breathing becomes shallow. Cortisol is released from the brain so that the survival mechanism sets in – "fight or flight."

Basically, we "download" every single negative event that occurs in our life. Some experience tragedy. We call that "Big T" tragedy. Examples of this are excessive childhood abuse, rape, incest, serious accidents, war-related experiences and so on. Others more commonly experience "Small T" tragedies: negative reminders from parents and other role models, emotional experiences in relationships, negative work experience, embarrassing childhood events, etc.

Whether you have experienced "Big T" or "Small T" events in your life, each event has changed your brain chemistry and left an imprint in your DNA. These add up and impact your thinking, your belief system, your attitude, your health, and more. When EFT is applied, the disruption in the energy system is released and the impact of these harmful memories changes from negative to neutral. When you recall the memory after the application of EFT Tapping, it is like watching a movie rather than reliving the event.

Here is a list of some of the most popular situations that have been transformed with the use of EFT Tapping:

- Addictions and Obsessions
- Allergy Relief/Allergies
- Asthma Relief
- Childhood Pain
- Fears and Phobias
- Health Concerns
- Insomnia/Sleep Problems
- Limiting Thoughts that may be blocking abundance, health and more
- Pain Management
- Painful Memories/Events
- PTSD (Post Traumatic Stress Disorder)
- Relationship Problems
- Tension Headaches and Migraine Headaches
- Trauma/Abuse
- Vision Issues
- Weight Loss/Eating Disorders

Now this may be "outside-the-box" for you, but I encourage you to at least check it out. Under the videos section on our site www.educationbeatsmedication.com we have included a few short but incredible videos which shows how one EFT session can be more beneficial than years of counseling or months of dietary changes and supplementing, etc.

We are emotional beings and those emotions can and will dictate our lives. We must take time to feed our spirit as we do our body. It took a long time for me, Dani, to take time for myself. Jack would always encourage me to do so and it would just make me mad. He just didn't realize how busy I was, how much I had to do and take care of! LOL

Yoga, meditation, prayer...there are so many things we can do. As my 'virtual' online world started to overwhelm me, taking a shower or a drive no longer cut it and I realized I had better find a great escape before I going completely mad so I started by shutting off our TV. Yes, we have survived without cable or satellite television for more than four years! It was the best thing we've done in a long time. We have Netflix and rent movies but we decide what we watch, listen to and allow in. Now, when I am at a friends or traveling and watch TV I am appalled to the point of disgusted at the commercials, the programming, the total manipulation and racket people are exposing themselves and their children to but years ago I was desensitized to it. Another thing always long for is nature, no cell phones, no internet, just me and the sound of the birds, wind and water. As I get "grounded" in the garden or go on a hike, all the troubles of the day just fade away. Jack, the boys and I look forward to white water rafting or camping to re-set our circadian rhythm (body clock). Unplugging from all the chaos and white noise helps us clear our thoughts, heck it helps me hear my thoughts, let go of so much that really does not matter and just be; in a state of love, gratitude and compassion.

Chapter 11: Hindsight's Always 20/20!

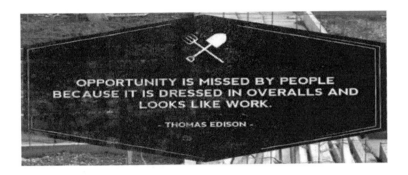

We hope to have expanded your horizons and opened your mind to a multitude of healing possibilities without completely overwhelming you! Wellness is so individual that it is impossible to come up with a "One size fits all" plan. You see, our goal was never to dictate to you exactly what to do...we do not know your diet, medications, beliefs, dis-eases, etc. and would not dare tell you what to do.   If you read the entire book and listened to the audios you've certainly gained enough to make a more informed decision for your health, to feel empowered and a bit more confident with the medical community, not in a bad way but in an aware way. It's all about implementing and staying committed to living a better quality of life for your children, for your spouse but most importantly, for yourself.

Even though we talk a lot about what to eat our understanding of inflammatory disease goes beyond diet. Prioritizing sleep, managing stress, breathing and incorporating plenty of mild to moderately-intense activity (and avoiding strenuous activity) into your day is also extremely important. This is why we included the chapter trivia and audios. Taking the holistic approach and in fact, if you ignore these lifestyle factors, you might completely undermine all of the effort you make with your diet.

Hindsight's always 20/20 is a phrase used to describe the fact that it is easy for us to be knowledgeable about an event after it has happened. Boy is that true yet knowing what we know now, neither of us would change a thing because every single circumstance, choice, direction and dead end, in retrospect, brought us to where we are today; a whole and healthy family unit. In hindsight we've spent the last 9 years becoming knowledgeable about options for overcoming dis-ease so we could share this knowledge and give direction to those searching for hope. *Against All Odds*, contains all the education we wish we had 9 years ago.

Having said this, if Jack were diagnosed with Sarcoidosis today he would go straight from the ENT that diagnosed him, to his MD for a blood draw to be sent to Immuno Laboratories for food intolerance testing! Even though food intolerances do not cause Sarcoidosis (as far as anyone knows) they do cause unwanted symptoms and tons of inflammation within the body, which complicate any disease.

An excerpt from Jeffrey Zaviks' book *Toxic Food Syndrome* says it best:

> "That is the sad truth about Toxic Food Syndrome. Fast-acting poisons like arsenic may take a few

minutes to kill their victims, while the poison of toxic food can subject its victims to decades of living death. What else would you call a life of constant pain, respiratory problems, digestive ailments, or fatigue?"

Instead of prednisone he would alter his diet by cutting out all dairy, processed foods, refined sugars and add supplements containing antioxidants and fucoidan. Every morning he would enjoy a green smoothie with superfoods like kale, spinach and berries and of course he would continue to drink 1/2oz per pound of filtered water at room temperature every day. Adding fresh lemon to flavor and help alkalize his body. Other than dietary changes Jack would have thermography every 6 months to monitor granulomas.

We are very thankful to have gone through such an experience and come out better people on the other side. Sarcoidosis threatened to steal our fairy tale lives and through what I refer to as "the slow erosion" we all started to wonder if it would succeed but we never let the doubt, misunderstanding and lack of direction hold us for long. Sure we had our days but we refused to allow it to become our life; fighting back with all our heart, mind and strength.

We encourage you to find something you love and do it for at least 15 minutes every day...walking, soak in hot tub, EFT, yoga, swimming, reading, painting, building model planes, gardening, meditation...JUST DO IT! You deserve 15 minutes reserved just for you every day. Do your best to get at least 6 hours of un-interrupted sleep every 24 hours. Your body needs this down time to repair and so does your mind. 8 hours a night is preferable. Sleep is tough when on prednisone: try a hot Epsom salt soak before bed. If your health allows, 20-30 minutes of walking everyday will do you wonders. Jack likes to ride his bike because it does not jar his knees. Rebounders are small trampolines which are excellent for helping to cleanse the lymph and activate every cell in your body. You do not need to jump, just bounce for 5-15 without your feet leaving the surface.

It takes 21 days to make or break a habit – if all of this at once is too much, pick one and start there. The goal is to live a better quality of life in complete wellness. Commit to a minimum of 90 days - It takes time and consistency.

After the first 30 days you may consider a cleanse or detox but be sure to seek a professional! I, Dani, am not a professional in anything and some of you may be ready for a cleanse from the start but many people are on serious medications, eat pour diets and I feel that taking the first 30 days to make these healthy adjustments will only help the cleanse be even more successful.

Continue to "clean up" your plate. Refer to foods to eat in Chapter 6 and recipes in Chapter 12. You may want to consult your physician before starting this healthier lifestyle but everything we share in this book have been used in conjunction with medical treatment.

Letting go of past pain, anger, resentments, blame, guilt, failures was also a huge part of Jack's ultimate healing. During his medical treatment he and I were going through some of our toughest years of marriage and sickness just intensified things. It was time for us to figure out how to love and appreciate each other rather than resent and blame. We each went through healing prayer sessions, leaned on friends who fought for us when we were ready to throw in the towel, went to a 4 day retreat which focused on processing through past events that held each of us back (it was NOT fun but very freeing).

I believe in a higher power, a creator who made everything on this planet to keep us healthy and whole; mind, body and spirit. Believing in something bigger than me gets me through the most difficult days and helps me find peace in the chaos. Through our healing journey over the last 9 years we've become aware of so many different ways to heal the mind, body and spirit. We continue our quest to gain knowledge. We keep an open mind. We include our kids in everything we do. We live out loud and believe that the universe gives us exactly what we ask for. It may not be what we expected but it does present itself, sometimes in the most awful packages.

Life is what we make it and dis-ease could just be an opening to marvelous things in your life. If you would have told Jack and I 10 years ago that we would be speaking at conferences, writing books, doing teleseminars, helping people all over the world and creating lifetime friendships because of Sarcoidosis...we would have laughed in your face (I, Dani, would have rolled my eyes ☺). But here we are and here you are. Do not pass up the opportunity to live a life free from the limitations of dis-ease or anything else.

You spent the money to get these resources, we are here to support and encourage you as well as everyone else in the "Surviving Sarcoidosis" community. Now it is up to you to take that next step. You may fall but we will help you get back up. You may lose hope but we will give you some of ours. You may be scared but what's the worst that could happen?

When Greg brought the antioxidants to the restaurant and said "What if it works?" Jack had nothing to lose and everything to gain, yet my spirit was challenged to think otherwise. "What if it doesn't?" At that time we were up a creek without a paddle, trying anything and everything to navigate and survive Sarcoidosis against all odds. Many times we spun in circles and ended up right back where we started but we never gave up.

What if Greg would not have offered his courage and belief? What if life happened, like it did for the guest on my radio show and Greg just did not show? Who knows where Jack would be right now. I know I never would have started a blog, a radio show and we never would have met Jacqueline, Morten, Rosa, Keith, Gail, Ken, Betty, Dianne, Kate, Deborah, John, Amy, Joe, Christina, Jaz, Emma, Martine, Sean, Marilyn, Zhenia, Mike and thousands of courageous people searching for lasting solutions. These are people we've been able to help because Greg first helped us. It is amazing how one single event can change the trajectory of 100's of lives. That day Greg started what we are now finishing...the book *Against All Odds* & *Education Beats Medication* audio series!

Remember when I told you it was time for a sabbatical well the time has come for us spur you into action! It's time, time to get up out of that recliner. This is your beginning; the first day of education beats medication for you. One day at a time you will overcome against all odds! You too have a story, one worth telling. It is not what you take but what you give in this life so celebrate the small stuff! Every day is worth savoring, every smile is worth giving and every breath is worth fighting for.

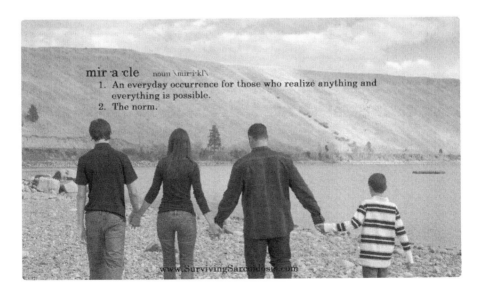

Because of Greg's' belief Jack and I are now helping people physically and financially. Our life really is a complete fairy tale. We have a story, a powerful story of hope and our persistence may just overcome conventional wisdom's resistance. One can only hope!

Your humbled and honored servants,

Jack & Dani Walker
The Snarky Sarkie and His Sassy Spouse!

Chapter 12: Resources, Recipes and Links

Be sure to email us your book receipt to access all the information and more on our site www.educationbeatsmedication.com

Documentaries to watch: (links to watch them for FREE)

This Beautiful Truth: http://youtu.be/wvzDHGLEUyw
What The Bleep Do We Know: http://youtu.be/ioONhpIJ-NY
The Gerson Miracle: http://youtu.be/sblixJI_oa4
The Endocannabinoids System: http://youtu.be/hHnQ-YAqAsA
Blue Gold: http://youtu.be/B1a3tjqQiBl

Toxins In Personal Care Products: http://www.ewg.org/ **or** www.skindeep.com

Hair Tissue Mineral Analysis:
http://drlwilson.com/do%20hair%20analysis.htm

Water Filtration:
http://h2o.educationbeatsmedication.com

Foods and Supplements:

Azure Standard – http://www.azurestandard.com/ great deals on organic, bulk foods and toxin-free products. Azure standard delivers to your town where you go pick it up at the drop off location.

Amazing Grass Green Superfoods – http://grass.educationbeatsmedication.com green superfoods supplements in all flavors

Fucoydon, Spectramaxx, Eternity – http://supplements.educationbeatsmedication.com These supplements are formulated in the USA by a network marketing company SISEL International but don't worry , there is no cost to become a customer and you get a 20% rebate to be used for future purchases – just save the welcome email with your account info. Be sure to choose preferred customer, then the country you are ordering in. You will find the supplements under the "Age Reversal" section. Fucoydon, Spectramaxx, Eternity are exclusively sold through manufacturers reps and not found in stores. Distributors pay a $20 fee to join and do not get any rebates. In full disclosure, every month 100% of commissions earned are gifted to foundations and charities which support the people with inflammatory disease.

Surviving Sarcoidosis Amazon Store – http://amazon.educationbeatsmedication.com books, movies, kitchen essentials and wellness supplements/supplies

Free Acid Alkaline Diet newsletter/recipes: http://diet.educationbeatsmedication.com

Audio Interviews: get a copy @ http://educationbeatsmedication.com All of these experts have free resources on their websites so even if you cannot get their services, go check out the free info.

1. **Surviving Sarcoidosis with Jack & Dani Walker**

2. **The Epigenetics Of Chronic Illness with Dr Michael Gruttadauria**

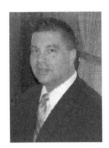 Specializing in Autistic Spectrum Disorders, Concussion/mTBI and Chronic Health Conditions http://beatautismnow.com Dr. Michael Gruttadauria is a graduate of NY Chiropractic College and is one of only 600 Board Certified Chiropractic Neurologists in the world. Best known for his application of this work to patients with Autism, Doctor. Download *Beat Autism Now* free @ www.beatautismnow.com

3. **Toxic Food Syndrome with Immunolabs Founder Jeffrey Zavik**

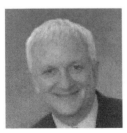 Immuno Laboratories in Fort Lauderdale, Florida, is widely recognized as one of the leading food and environmental allergy testing facilities in the world. Since its inception in 1978, the company has conducted over 29 million food sensitivity tests. To download Jeffrey Zaviks' book *Toxic Food Syndrome* free @ www.sendmethefreebook.com

4. The Lost Art Of Cleansing with Laurel Sander

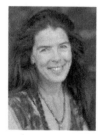

http://windspiritmedicine.com/ Laurel Sander has 25 years of experience in the Healing Arts and Holistic Medicine; Doctor of Oriental Medicine, D.O.M. (NM), Nationally Certified Acupuncturist, L. Ac. (NCCAOM, NM, UT, and OR) Massage Therapist, Tui Na Spinal Alignment, Chinese Herbologist, Kinesiologist, Reflexology, Energy Medicine/Shamanic Tracking, Nutritionist and Whole Body Medicine. Author of Hope To Heal Cleanse, a step-by-step in home cleanse course complete with DVD; get a copy @ http://www.hopetoheal.us/

5. How To Cleanse Safely with Dr. Richard Powell

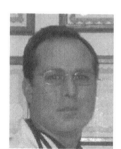

Doctor Richard Powell, N.D, OMD, CAc, Ph.D. and co-host of "The Medical Insiders" radio show with Dani Walker. He has been practicing and utilizing alternative medicine for the past 28 years. Dr Richard Powell is a Naturopathic and Oriental Medical Doctor, Life and Wellness Coach, Acupuncturist and published author.

6. Allergies & Toxicity with Dr Delrae

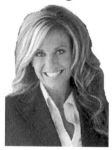

https://www.drdelraedetox.com/ Doctor Delrae is a Chiropractor. After her own health struggles she developed the DrDelRae Detox and Weight Loss System: detoxing at a cellular level, jump-start your bodies fat-burning furnace and providing muscle with high quality protein to burn fat. Be sure to download her free ebook.

7. Powered By Green Smoothies with Sergei Boutenko

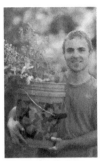

http://sergeiboutenko.com/ or www.rawfamily.com Sergei Boutenko is a 28 years old adventurer, author, videographer, and lover of life. Sergei and his family have been inspiring people to add greens to their diet and transform their health for 25+ years. Pioneers in the raw food, green smoothies movement.

8. Toxic Times How It's Made with Tom Mower

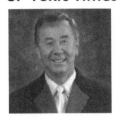

Thomas Mower Sr., Chairman of SISEL International is a leader in the field of nutritional and personal care products and natural cosmetics for the last 30 years.

9. What Is Thermography with Jeannie Nelson, CTT, NTP

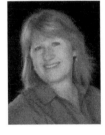

www.medicalthermographynw.com Jeannie Nelson of Medical Thermography Northwest and Southwest is a Certified Thermography Technician and Certified Nutritional Therapy Practitioner.

10. EFT - Mind Over Matter with Life Coach Marla Tabaka

Marla is The Million-Dollar Mindset Coach and specializes in coaching women business owners who are ready to embrace their full potential in life and business. You can schedule a free 20 minute EFT session with Marla at http://www.marlatabaka.com/eft-tapping/

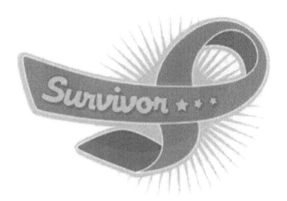

Sarcoidosis, Research, Foundations, Support and More:

Sarcoidosis Center List of Sarcoidosis Centers, Addresses, and Sarcoidosis Info: http://sarcoidcenter.com
Sarcoidosis Statistics:
http://www.lung.org/assets/documents/publications/solddc-chapters/sarcoidosis.pdf
FAQ's About Sarcoidosis: http://www.sarcoid-network.org/FAQ/faq-disease.php
Epidemiology of Sarcoidosis:
http://www.ildcare.eu/Downloads/artseninfo/Sarcoidosis/Chapter%202%20Epidemiology%20of%20sarcoidosis.pdf
Western medicine options for Sarcoidosis:
http://my.clevelandclinic.org/disorders/sarcoidosis/hic_sarcoidosis_treatment_options.aspx
National Jewish Medical and Research Center:
http://www.nationaljewish.org/
Sarcoidosis Clinical Trials/Research Studies:
http://www.nhlbi.nih.gov/health/dci/Diseases/sarc/sar_links.html
WASOG World Association of Sarcoidosis and Other Granulomas Diseases: http://www.wasog.org/

National Heart, Lung, Blood Institute (NHLBI) Sarcoidosis Facts: http://www.gradslung.org/sarcoidosis.html

Support Groups, Forums and Foundations:

UK Sarcoidosis Support: http://sa-uk.org/
Sarcoidosis Ning: http://sarcoidosis.ning.com One of the first support forums I found!
Sarcoidosis Reach For A Cure facebook group: https://www.facebook.com/pages/Sarcoidosis-Reach-for-a-Cure/299962673213
Worldwide Directory Of Sarcoidosis Support Groups: http://www.sarcoidosisonlinesites.com/support%20groups.htm
Sarcoidosis Registry: http://www.snaregistry.org/
Sarcoidosis Resource Center: http://www.nsrc-global.net/
Oregon Sarcoidosis Network: http://sarcoidosisnetwork.org/
Foundation For Sarcoidosis Research: www.stopsarcoidosis.org
Interstitial Lung Disease Australia: http://www.lungfoundation.com.au
Irish Sarcoidosis Support Network: http://www.isarc.ie/
Life and Breath Foundation: http://www.lifeandbreath.org/

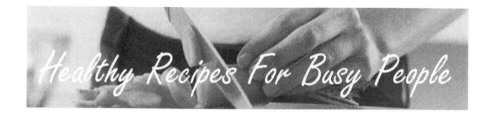

Healthy Recipes For Busy People

GREEN SMOOTHIE RECIPES – from rawfamily.com

Basic Balance
1 mango
1 cup kale
1 cup water
Yields 1 quart

Rocket Fuel Smoothie
2 cups green or red
seedless grapes
3 golden kiwis, peeled
1 ripe orange, peeled,
seeds removed
1 small leaf of aloe vera,
with skin
5 leaves red leaf lettuce
2 cups water
Yields 2 quarts

Morning Zing Smoothie
4:½ bunch dandelion
greens
2 stalks celery
½ inch fresh gingerroot
2 peaches
½ pineapple
Yields 2 quarts

Parsley Passion Smoothie
1 bunch fresh parsley
1 cucumber, peeled
1 Fuji apple

Party in Your Mouth Green Smoothie
1 small pineapple, cored
1 large mango, peeled
½ head romaine lettuce
½ inch fresh ginger root
Yields 2 quarts

Pack A Punch: add 2 TBSP aloe vera and/or the Green Superfoods powder to any of these smoothies. You can add the Fucoydon and Spectramaxx too. Flax oil, hemp seeds, flax seeds or chia seeds are great too.

These all yield 1 quart. Drink throughout the day. We refrigerate in glass kerr jars for up to 48 hours.

SET IT AND FORGET IT CROCKPOT RECIPES: Jack and I are realists – even though RAW is best, time is precious. Having a crockpot saves so much time and ensures that we have a pretty healthy meal every night. Just add ingredients and go.

Coconut Curry Chicken

INGREDIENTS:
1 can coconut milk
2 Tbsp raw grass-fed but
2 Tbsp curry powder
2 lbs chicken
2 cups frozen broccoli

DIRECTIONS:
1. Pour coconut milk in crock-pot.
2. Add butter and curry powder.
3. Add chicken and top with broccoli.
4. Cook on low for 4-6 hours.
5. ENJOY!

Cinnamon Raisin Oatmeal

INGREDIENTS:
2 cups organic almond or coconut milk
1 Tbsp honey
1 tsp cinnamon
1 Tbsp organic brown sugar or 2 packets

DIRECTIONS:
Grease crock-pot with coconut oil.
Add all ingredients, mix together.
Cook on LOW for 5-6 hours
ENJOY!

stevia
1 cup gluten-free oats or steel cut oats
1 cup chopped apple (I left the peel on)
1/2 cup chopped walnuts
1/2 cup raisins

Pesto Polenta:

3 tablespoons melted butter or olive oil	1/4 tsp paprika
6 cups boiling water	2 c cornmeal
2 teaspoons kosher or sea salt	2 TBSP pesto

Directions:
Coat Crock Pot with 1 tablespoon olive oil. Measure remaining ingredients; add to slow cooker with remaining butter or olive oil. Stir well; cover and cook on low for 5 to 8 hours (2 to 3 hours on high), stirring occasionally. Once polenta has thickened cover top with sliced zucchini, and onions, then marinara sauce and cook in crockpot for another 1 to 2 hours on low. Let cool for 30 minutes and top with feta.

Dani's Favorite Vegetarian Chili

1 package pinto beans or mixed beans	1 teaspoon cumin
1 tablespoon olive oil	1 teaspoon sea salt
3 medium yellow onions	1 quart vegetable broth
3 cloves garlic	2 - 28-ounce can crushed tomatoes
2 carrots finely chopped	3 tablespoons catsup
1 ½ tablespoons chili powder	½ tablespoon cocoa powder
2 zucchini finely chopped	

DIRECTIONS:

The night before making the chili, rinse and cover the beans with water in a bowl. Soak overnight at room temperature. Prepare the fresh ingredients (this can be done early and kept in the refrigerator): Dice onions, carrots, zucchini about 10 hours before serving, discard the liquid on the beans and place the beans in a large slow cooker. Transfer all ingredients to the slow cooker with the beans. Cover with vegetable broth and crushed tomatoes. Cook on low for 10-12 hours. When ready to serve, garnish with green onions and plain Greek yogurt.

SIMPLE SALADS AND DRESSINGS:

Italian Dressing

1 ¼ c oil (olive oil, sesame or flax oil) (filtered ☺)

1 c water

¾ c lemon juice (fresh squeezed)

1 ½ t sea salt

1 ½ t garlic powder powder

1 ½ T onion

1 T *fresh or dried Basil Parsley

2 T *fresh or dried

Mix all ingredients and shake.

*When using fresh basil and parsley - use a blender or cuisine art to integrate herbs.

Orange Basil Vinaigrette (this is the most requested recipe at Calderas)

1 cup fresh Basil

½ cup white wine vinegar

4 Oranges

1 ½ cups Olive Oil

Juice the oranges and put all ingredients in a cuisanart, blend and enjoy! Saves up to 4 weeks in fridge. You can also add 1 TBSP honey to sweeten.

Berry Summer Salad
Ingredients
8 cups mixed salad greens   2 cups fresh blueberries
1/2 cup crumbled Gorgonzola or blue cheese
1/4 cup chopped and toasted walnuts or pecans

Toss together first 4 ingredients; drizzle with desired amount of vinaigrette, tossing gently to coat.

Beet and Goat Cheese Arugula Salad
Ingredients
1/4 cup balsamic vinegar   1/2 avocado, cubed
3 tablespoons shallots, thinly sliced   1 tablespoon honey
1/3 cup extra-virgin olive oil
Salt and ground black pepper
6 medium beets, cooked and quartered
6 cups fresh arugula or salad greens
1/2 cup walnuts, toasted, coarsely chopped
1/4 cup dried cranberries or dried cherries
3 ounces soft fresh goat cheese, coarsely crumbled

Directions:
Line a baking sheet with foil. Preheat the oven to 450 degrees F.
Whisk the vinegar, shallots, and honey in a medium bowl to blend. Gradually whisk in the oil. Season the vinaigrette, to taste, with salt and pepper. Toss the beets in a small bowl

with enough dressing to coat. Place the beets on the prepared baking sheet and roast until the beets are slightly caramelized, stirring occasionally, about 12 minutes. Set aside and cool.

Toss the arugula, walnuts, and cranberries in a large bowl with enough vinaigrette to coat. Season the salad, to taste, with salt and pepper. Mound the salad atop 4 plates. Arrange the beets around the salad. Sprinkle with the avocado and goat cheese, and serve.

Spinach Salad (another favorite from our family restaurant: Calderas)
Ingredients   toss all ingredients in bowl and enjoy!
2 fresh cups spinach   4 TBSP walnuts
1 TBSP dried cranberries ½ orange, peeled and chunked
2-3 TBSP feta cheese
Orange Basil Vinaigrette (recipe above)

Cilantro Cole Slaw
Ingredients
1 head cabbage (green or purple)   3 carrots shredded
1 cup chopped chives   1 c chopped cilantro
1 TBSP lemon juice or apple cider vinegar
1/2 cup soy free mayonnaise   1 tsp dill seed
Salt and pepper to taste
toss all ingredients together till mixed – best after setting for 1-2 hours

Quinoa Lentil Salad

Ingredients

1/2 cup quinoa

1 1/4 cups water, plus 2 cups

1/2 cup lentils

1/4 teaspoon garlic powder

2 green onions chopped

2 tablespoons red wine vinegar

1 tablespoon chopped fresh cilantro leaves

1 lime, zested

1/4 cup vegetable oil

1 teaspoon Dijon mustar

black pepper

Kosher salt

Directions:

1. Put the quinoa in a sieve and rinse in cold water. In a large pan with lid, add the rinsed quinoa and 1 1/4 cups water, bring to boil and put on simmer for 10 minutes. Let it sit for 2 minutes then stir. Quinoa should be tender enough to eat, but with a little "pop" upon biting.
2. Put the lentils in a sieve and rinse in cold water. In a saucepan, simmer the lentils in 2 cups water until the lentils are tender, but not mushy, about 30 minutes. Drain and cool.
3. In a small bowl, whisk the mustard and vinegar together, and drizzle in the oil to make an emulsion. Add the garlic powder, lime zest, and salt, and pepper, to taste.
4. To assemble the salad: In a medium salad bowl, mix the quinoa, lentils, green onions, and chopped cilantro. Top the salad with the dressing, toss to coat and serve.

Olive Oil Butter

Yeilds: 1 ½ lbs
Blend: 2 tsp unflavored gelatin   1 c hot water
Add: 1 ½ cup olive oil, 1 tsp salt and ¼ tsp turmeric
Blend until smooth. Chill in glass container 30 min - 1 hr
Variation: Garlic butter - add 2-3 cloves garlic or ½ t garlic
powder to gelatin and water

HEALTHY SNACKS:

Zucchini Parmesan Chips - I double this recipe

2 medium zucchini (about 1 pound total)
1 tablespoon olive oil
1/4 cup freshly grated Parmesan (3/4-ounce)
1/4 cup panko or cracker crumbs
1/8 teaspoon sea salt
Freshly ground black pepper

Directions:
Preheat the oven to 450 degrees F. Coat a baking sheet
with olive oil.
Slice the zucchini into 1/4-inch thick rounds. In a medium
bowl, toss the zucchini with the oil. In a small bowl,
combine the Parmesan, panko, salt, and a few turns of
pepper. Dip each round into the Parmesan mixture, coating
it evenly on both sides, pressing the coating on to stick, and
place in a single layer on the prepared baking sheet. Bake
the zucchini rounds until browned and crisp, 25 to 30
minutes. Remove with spatula. Serve immediately.

Kale or Chard Chips (can use beet greens too)
1 bunch kale, chard or beet greens cut in 3x3" chips
Toss in bowl with 1 TBSP olive oil, sea salt and pepper
Bake on 225 - 20-25 minutes (until crips)   may need to
check and flip after 10 minutes

Sweet Potato Fries
4 sweet potatoes, peeled and cut into long French fries

1/4 cup olive oil	1/2 teaspoon ground black pepper
1 tsp steak seasoning	1/2 teaspoon garlic powder
1/4 teaspoon salt	1/4 teaspoon paprika

Directions:
Place sweet potato fries into a large bowl, drizzle with 1/4
cup olive oil, and toss to coat. Mix steak seasoning, black
pepper, garlic powder, salt, and paprika in a separate small
bowl until thoroughly combined. Use your left hand to toss
fries with olive oil as you sprinkle the seasoning mixture
over them with your right hand.
Heat 1 tablespoon olive oil in a large skillet over medium
heat and place sweet potato pieces into the hot oil. Cover
skillet, pan-fry for 5 minutes; uncover and turn fries. Place
cover back over fries and cook 5 more minutes; continue
turning fries and covering until sweet potatoes are tender,
about 10 more minutes.

Easy Healthy Cookie Dough
To make your cookie dough, just mix up two soft bananas
with a cup of dry oats, adding more oats if it seems too
runny.

That is literally the entire recipe. Once your dough is mixed, just dollop it onto a greased cookie sheet and bake at 350 degrees for about 15 minutes. When they're done, you'll have some healthy snacks that are easy to eat on the go. If you want to customize the flavor, you can sprinkle in some chocolate chips, cinnamon, craisins, raisins, ground flax, coconut, blueberries or pretty much anything else.

Homemade Hot/Cold Wrap (stores sell these for $40)
Take a thick, long athletic sock and fill it with any rice you have. Fold and sow the top shut. Done! You can put it in the freezer for an instant and comfortable cold pack or microwave it for 2 minutes and use as a hot pad.

Get creative and try new things! Food is fun and real food is amazing...we will share new recipes often so be sure to open emails from life@eduationbeatsmedication.com and let us know of any awesome recipes you are using as well.

Your partners in surviving against all odds,
Jack and Dani Walker

About The Author:

"Wellness is the connection of paths between knowledge & action." Dani Walker

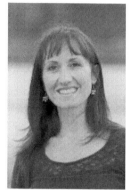

Dani Walker is an author, founder of Education Beats Medication, permission to think outside the prescription for total wellness & Mompreneur, best known for her international radio show "The Medical Insider".

She demands that people question everything & spends much of her time relentlessly searching for the "outside the box" knowledge and wisdom to manifest total wellness in her life and others.

Dani is the oldest of 5, raised in small town America by her single Mom who exemplified tenacity, compassion and strength. Her husband Jack's diagnosis spurred her to become a "medical private investigator" but she relentlessly continues her work as many loved ones struggle with seemingly incurable diseases.

A self-professed "Jack of all trades, master of none" Dani brings her circle of influential people together to help you turn your passions and/or misfortunes into profits & live a life free from the limitations of disease & debt. Meet Dani at www.daniwalker.com

References:

0. List Autoimmune Diseases http://www.aarda.org/autoimmune-information/list-of-diseases/
1. National Heart, Lung and Blood Institute. Diseases and Conditions Index. Sarcoidosis: Causes.February 2009. http://www.nhlbi.nih\.gov/health/dci/Diseases/sarc/sar_causes.html.
2. Guz, A. (1997). Brain, breathing and breathlessness. Respiration Physiology. 109, 197-204.
3. Computing Toxic Chemicals, July 18, 2013 http://www.sciencedaily.com/releases/2013/07/130718101337.htm
4. J Gerontol A Biol Sci Med Sci. 2007 Nov;62(11):1199-203. http://www.ncbi.nlm.nih.gov/pubmed/18000138
5. Tumor necrosis factor-alpha inhibitor treatment for sarcoidosis http://www.ncbi.nlm.nih.gov/pmc/articles/PMC2643111/
6. Scott H Beegle, Kerry Barba, Romel Gobunsuy, and Marc A Judson Drug Des Devel Ther. 2013; 7: 325–338. 2013 April 12. doi: 10.2147/DDDT.S31064 Current and emerging pharmacological treatments for sarcoidosis: a review
7. Curr Opin Pulm Med. 2010 Sep. Oxidative stress and antioxidants in interstitial lung disease. http://www.ncbi.nlm.nih.gov/pubmed/20592594
8. Respir Med. 2009 Sep;103(9):1245-56. doi: 10.1016/j.rmed.2009.04.014. Epub 2009 May 22. Oxidative stress in the pathogenesis of diffuse lung diseases: a review. http://www.ncbi.nlm.nih.gov/pubmed/19464864
9. Sarcoidosis Vasc Diffuse Lung Dis. 2008 Dec;25(2):140-2.Improvement of cardiac sympathetic nerve function in sarcoidosis. http://www.ncbi.nlm.nih.gov/pubmed/19382533
10. Respir Med. 2009 Mar;103(3):364-72. doi: 10.1016/j.rmed.2008.10.007. Epub 2008 Nov 17. Antioxidant status associated with inflammation in sarcoidosis: a potential role for antioxidants.
11. Curr Med Res Opin. 2008 Jun;24(6):1651-7. Epub 2008 May 9. Levels of paraoxonase, an index of antioxidant defense, in patients with active sarcoidosis. http://www.ncbi.nlm.nih.gov/pubmed/18474147
12. Tumor Necrosis Factor alpha - http://www.ncbi.nlm.nih.gov/pmc/articles/PMC2643111/
13. Do H, Pyo S, Sohn EH. Suppression of iNOS expression by fucoidan is mediated by regulation of p38 MAPK, JAK/STAT, AP-1 and IRF-1, and depends on up-regulation of scavenger receptor B1 expression in TNF-alpha- and IFN-gamma-stimulated C6 glioma cells. J Nutr Biochem. 2009 Jul 1.
14. Phytomedicine, 2005 Jun, 12(6-7):445-52, "The effect of turmeric extracts on inflammatory mediator production"
15. Chuang et al. Quercetin is equally or more effective than resveratrol in attenuating tumor necrosis factor-alpha-mediated inflammation and insulin resistance in primary human adipocytes. Am J Clin Nutr 92:1511-21 (2010).
16. Cancer Detect Prev, 2000, 24(1):91-9, "A new concept of tumor promotion by tumor necrosis factor-alpha, and cancer preventive agents (-)-epigallocatechin gallate and green tea--a review"
17. Sandoval et al. Cat's claw inhibits TNFalpha production and scavenges free radicals: role in cytoprotection. Free Radic Biol Med 29(1):71-8 (2000).
18. BioFactors, 2008, 32(1-4):179-183, "Functions of coenzyme Q_{10} in inflammation and gene expression"
19. Powerful electrolyte - Jackson, William R. (1993). Humic, Fulvic and Microbial Balance: Organic Soil Conditioning, 329. Evergreen, Colorado: Jackson Research Center.
20. Mineral complexes in fulvic may serve as electrodes – Rashid, M.A. (1985). Geochemistry of marine humic substances. New York: Springer-Verlag.

21. Free radical – Senesi, N. (1990) Analytica Chmica Acta, 232, 51-75. Amsterdam, The Netherlands: Elsevier.

22. Williams, S. T. (1963). Are antibiotics produced in soil? Pedobiologia, 23, 427-435.

23. proteins, DNA, RNA – Khristeva, L.A., Soloche, K.I., Dynkina, R.L., Kovalenko, V.E., & Gorobaya, A.I. (1967). Influence of physiologically active substances of soil humus and fertilizers on nucleic acid metabolism, plant growth and subsequent quality of the seeds. Humus et Planta, 4, 272-276.

24. Sharma OP. Vitamin D, calcium, and sarcoidosis. Chest 1996; 109:535.

25. Cell elongation - Poapst, P.A., & Schnitzer, M. (1971). Fulvic acid and adventitious root formation. Soil Biology and Biochemistry, 3, 215-219.

26. Guohua Cao*, Helaine M. Alessio†, Richard G. Cutler Oxygen-radical absorbance capacity assay for antioxidants

27. Trace Mineral Poor Food/Soil Depletion http://unicef.org/nutrition/index_hidden_hunger.html

28. Hirayasu H, Yoshikawa Y, Tsuzuki S, Fushiki T. Sulfated polysaccharides derived from dietary seaweeds increase the esterase activity of a lymphocyte tryptase, granzyme A. J Nutr Sci Vitaminol (Tokyo). 2005 Dec;51(6):475-7.

29. Irhimeh MR, Fitton JH, Lowenthal RM.Fucoidan ingestion increases the expression of CXCR4 on human CD34+ cells. Exp Hematol. 2007 Jun;35(6):989-94.

30. Jean-François Deux; Anne Meddahi-Pellé; Alain F. Le Blanche; Laurent J. Feldman; Sylvia Colliec-Jouault; Françoise Brée; Frank Boudghène; Jean-Baptiste Michel; Didier Letourneur (2002). Low Molecular Weight Fucoidan Prevents Neointimal Hyperplasia in Rabbit Iliac Artery In-Stent Restenosis Model (PDF). Arteriosclerosis, Thrombosis, and Vascular Biology. 22:1604.

31. Aisa Y, Miyakawa Y, Nakazato T, Shibata H, Saito K, Ikeda Y, Kizaki M. Fucoidan induces apoptosis of human HS-sultan cells accompanied by activation of caspase-3 and down-regulation of ERK pathways. American Journal of Hematology. 2005 Jan;78 (1): 7–14.

32. Maruyama H, Tamauchi H, Hashimoto M, Nakano T. Antitumor activity and immune response of Mekabu fucoidan extracted from Sporophyll of Undaria pinnatifida. In Vivo 2003; 17(3):245-249.

33. Do H, Pyo S, Sohn EH. Suppression of iNOS expression by fucoidan is mediated by regulation of p38 MAPK, JAK/STAT, AP-1 and IRF-1, and depends on up-regulation of scavenger receptor B1 expression in TNF-alpha- and IFN-gamma-stimulated C6 glioma cells. J Nutr Biochem. 2009 Jul 1. [Epub ahead of print]

34. Luo D, Zhang Q, Wang H, et al. Fucoidan protects against dopaminergic neuron death in vivo and in vitro. Eur J Pharmacol. 2009 Sep 1;617(1-3):33-40.

35. Janet Hellen Fitton Published online 2011 September 30. doi: 10.3390/md9101731 Therapies from Fucoidan; Multifunctional Marine Polymers http://www.ncbi.nlm.nih.gov/pmc/articles/PMC3210604/

36. by MT Borra - 2005 - Cited by 502 - Related articles J Biol Chem. 2005 Apr 29;280(17):17187-95. Epub 2005 Mar 4. www.ncbi.nlm.nih.gov/pubmed/15749705

37. Antioxidant Activity and Protective Effect on DNA Cleavage of Resveratrol R. Acquaviva, A. Russo, A. Campisi, V. Sorrenti, C. Giacomo, M.L. Barcellona, M. Avitabile, A. Vanella Journal of Food Science (impact factor: 1.66). 07/2006; 67(1):137 - 141. DOI:10.1111/j.1365-2621.2002.tb11373.x

38. Resveratrol exerts its neuroprotective effect by modulating mitochondrial dysfunctions associated cell death during cerebral ischemia; Seema Yousuf, Fahim Atif, Muzamil Ahmad, Nasrul Hoda

39. Memorial Sloan-Kettering Cancer Center: "Resveratrol."

40. Van der Spuy, W.J. Nutrition Research Reviews, Sept. 22 2009

41. Wilson, L., Nutritional Balancing and Hair Mineral Analysis, L.D. Wilson Consultants, Inc., 1991, 1998, 2005, 2010.

42. United States Environmental Protection Agency, Toxic Trace Metals in Mammalian Hair and Nails, EPA-600 4.79-049, August 1979